Natural Solutions

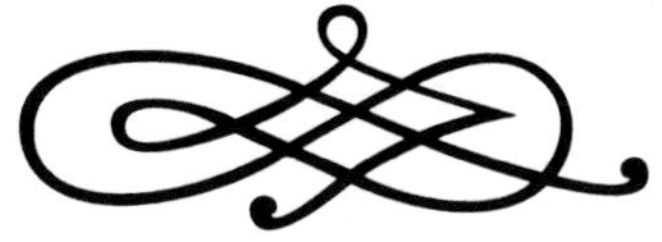

*"To every thing, there is a season,
and a time for every purpose
under the heaven"*

Ecclesiastes 3,1

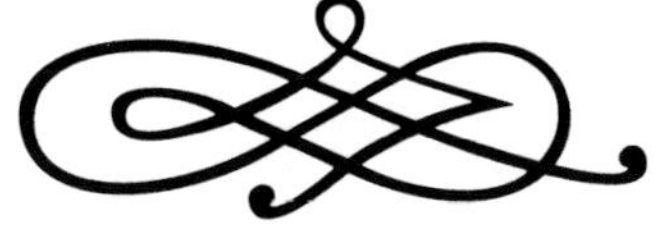

Natural Solutions

Women's Health Conditions

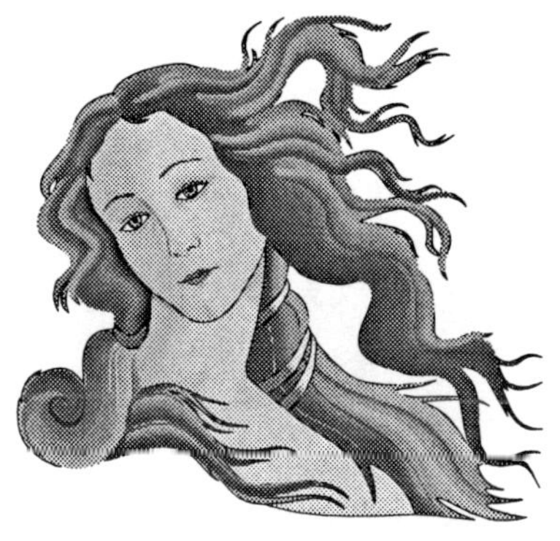

Ann Lisette Wesso
Holistic Health Practitioner
Clinical Hypnotherapist
Nutritional Counselor

Published by:
MoonRose Enterprises
8392 Capricorn Way #47
San Diego, California 92126

DISCLAIMER: This book is designed as a guide to inform, enlighten, encourage and empower women during crucial times in their life. It is not intended to diagnose ailments nor to be used as a substitute for professional medical care and/or treatment. Because there are always risks involved in anything, the author and publisher are not responsible for any adverse consequences or effects resulting from use of any information contained in this guide. If someone is unwilling to accept responsibility for making their own choices, then please do not read this. In case of serious illness be sure to consult a doctor or the professional heath care provider of your choice.

Layout and Graphics by: Signature Press

ISBN 0-9719447-1-7
Printed in the United States of America

Library of Congress Control
Number: 2002107800

Published by:
MoonRose Enterprises
8392 Capricorn Way #47
San Diego, California 92126
Email: Alwesso@aol.com

Dedicated to my Mother
Who did it naturally!
And whose spirit, love and wisdom
Have guided me all my life.

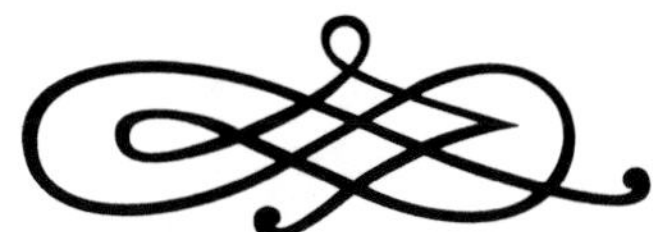

About the Author

Ann Lisette Wesso, a former corporate executive, is now the owner and founder of her own consulting company. Ann educates and counsels people on how to achieve more balance, peace and harmony in their lives on all levels: physical, mental, emotional, and spiritual. As a Mind-Body-Spirit Counselor, Ann addresses all areas of growth. She is trained as a Clinical Hypnotherapist, Holistic Health Practitioner, Nutritional Counselor, Master Practitioner of Neuro Linguistic Programming, Time Line Therapy™ Master Practitioner, Certified Trainer, Meditation Teacher, and Spiritual Counselor.

She is a professional member of the American Board of Hypnotherapy, the American Board of Neuro Linguistic Programming, Time Line Therapy Association™, and the American Association of Nutritional Consultants. She's a founding member of a wellness group in her community. Her experience includes consulting at Scripps Center for Executive Health in San Diego on stress management, and she has experience leading various support groups. In addition, she's worked at Deepak Chopra's Center for Mind-Body Healing and the Golden Door Spa.

Ann provides lifestyle coaching and guidance to clients in the areas of stress mastery, healing, career, emotional and spiritual growth and change. She leads support groups, teaches meditation, and facilitates seminars and workshops. This guide can stand on its own, and is also part of a program to educate women about the many natural and healthy solutions to women's health issues, including PMS, hormone replacement, perimenopause, menopause, and many other conditions. This guide is intended to help teach all women to understand the needs of their ever-changing bodies. Remedies and solutions suggested are safe, easy, natural, and women at any age can benefit from this information.

If you have questions, comments or experiences you might like to share, please contact Ann at alwesso@aol.com.

Preface

Many of you may be wondering why I wrote this book. My original intention was to have information for a seminar. I wished to do that seminar because as I was approaching mid-life, and I wanted to avoid the physical and emotional problems I'd been fighting all my life. I could have been the original PMS Poster Girl. My body had a mind of it's own and provided me a vast learning ground. Moodiness, bloating, cramps, weight gain, fibrocystic breasts, headaches, pain, and more. This was my life-long learning ground, and my desire was to lighten my load.

Various pharmaceutical drugs and hormones were prescribed over the years. The hormones were the worst of all for me. Birth control pills were out of the question because of numerous side effects and weight gain. As for the other drugs, which went from tranquilizers to mood stabilizers to water pills, the experience was incredible! Some helped but most didn't. Some had terrible side effects. Some made me a zombie and some made me hyper. I decided these did not work well for me, and I certainly did not want to be drugged through my transitional years.

Researching this book enlightened me. I realized how much I didn't know, plus I learned that there was more than one hormone that affected my health. It was a blessing that I accumulated this information when I did. Why, you may ask? Other than the obvious ones, which were to prevent my suffering and find out what other alternatives I might use in place of drugs, what was the blessing? I am not a promoter or believer in pharmaceutical drugs and yet, I realize there can be benefit in them for some people. In any case, the result was that this text provided me encouragement and a personal resource to refer to when I developed a breast tumor a couple years later.

The short version of this complicated story, is that I woke up one morning with a very large breast tumor on the inside of my right breast. It was extremely painful and, no doubt, a more dramatic manifestation of the fibrocystic breast condition I suffered with throughout my life. At the time, I did not have any medical insurance and was steeped in holistic approaches. Not only was I steeped in holistic approaches, I believed in them!

The journey through my awareness and eventual healing of the breast tumor is a topic for another book. Yet, after visiting my doctor, who's educated and experienced opinion was that it was breast cancer, and having a sonogram and determining that it was a solid breast tumor, I decided on a different course of action than traditional medicine.

This was not an "accepted" approach by my doctor or other medical professionals or even personal friends. I discovered their fears and traditional belief systems were what they referred to more often than supporting my desire to take care of myself naturally. My best supporter and angel was my mother, who totally trusted in my choice of action, or non-action as the case maybe, and always listened to me with love and compassion. I strive to be like her in my counseling work. She was my Guardian Angel on earth.

I used all natural, non-invasive techniques and products. A Naturopath friend helped me find the best homeopathics, encouraged my non-medical approach, and influenced me not to get caught up in the "fear." The most difficult aspect of it all, was to go against traditional practices. I included many alternatives in my healing, including yoga, meditation, diet, herbs, homeopathics, castor oil packs, visualization, and most especially, my angels, prayers, and changing my mind. My inner spiritual guidance was my best resource. God was with me the entire journey, and let me assure you, it was not an easy one. God did not get off without a lot of criticism, anger, and frustration during the process. However, in the end, I came to believe that God and my Faith, which is within each of us, is the true source of all my good.

The result is what matters. The result is that I no longer have a breast tumor. It was eliminated within two months and I am still living, and very happy and healthy, I might add. My doctor said I was "lucky." The truth is that I was proactive in my own healing and decision making, and I completely *believed in my choices.*

My prayer is that this guide is a resource for anyone seeking to find information, alternatives, or natural solutions to any health condition. I believe the "key" is to seek peace of mind in whatever form of healing you choose and to trust your inner guidance.

Ann Wesso
March, 2002

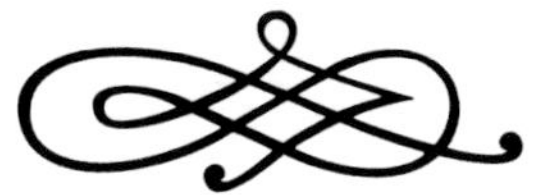

Acknowledgements

What I have written is a result of my life experiences and physical challenges from childhood through adulthood. Though it would be difficult to thank all those who've influenced me along the way, I would like to mention a few. For any omission, it is unintentional, so please forgive me. I acknowledge and thank those people who have assisted me with inspiration and support in preparing this text.

My mother who has always been my best friend and supporter.

To my brother Bill, who always told me to focus on one thing at a time.

To Yogananda for his inspirational wisdom and teachings especially those found in his book, *Scientific Healing Affirmations.*

To all my good friends, you know who you are, who have supported me in my goal to complete this book.

To David, a Naturopath guide and teacher, who taught me so much about health and how to trust my common sense and intuition over intellect.

To Laura, my Supervisor at Scripps, who has always expressed confidence in my abilities.

To my teachers, especially those who assisted me in Holistic Health, Hypnotherapy, Nutrition, Neuro Linguistic Programming, Meditation, Spirituality, and more.

To Kathy, owner of Signature Press, who consistently encouraged me to publish and improve on this book as well as her assistant Diana for providing additional ideas and suggestions.

To my grandmother, Mimi, for being so determined and strong and passing that on to me.

To my favorite authors who provided on-going inspiration when I needed it most.

To my Angels and Guides for inspiring my thoughts and dreams and giving me the courage to complete this book.

Table of Contents

Table of Contents (Continued)

Introduction

My Goal is to:

- *help women be more in touch with their bodies,*
- *assist them in making truly informed choices about their health and well-being,*
- *educate on the many natural solutions available to women, and*
- *change our perspective towards menopause as a normal, natural transition.*

I am a very young and vital woman fifty years old and suffered with premenstrual symptoms (PMS) most of my life, in fact, since I started having periods at age eleven. I went to so many doctors through the years and got so many conflicting opinions, I ended up confused about what to do and pretty much started following my own intuition. Not only that, but I was never able to use the drugs that were prescribed. They just never seemed to work for me. Now that I'm entering, and quite honestly, have been at perimenopause for awhile, I wanted to know the truth about all this, as well as PMS, menopause, osteoporosis, heart disease, and so much more.

First of all, I must say that women in America do not understand their bodies very well. In fact, we don't understand women's health issues because we have not been intelligently informed, and unfortunately, many doctors and health professionals haven't either. You can find information about PMS, perimenopause and menopause almost anywhere, except from your doctor. With all due respect to the medical profession, doctors are not taught much about natural remedies, nutrition, herbs, or even stress management and relaxation techniques. All of these are crucial for your best health.

This guide will inform you of the additional solutions available for various women's conditions, including PMS, perimenopause and menopause. There are many other solutions not included in this text, however, I hope that what is provided here will be a beginning of your on-going education. For those of you who have wondered if you have a choice other than drugs and/or hormone replacement, I am here to assure you that *you do have a choice!*

There are mountains of books, magazine and newspaper articles, interviews, and more about women's health issues, and thank goodness it's happening. Ten years ago, it was much more difficult to find the information. The question might now become, what should we believe? What will work for me? The new found popularity and controversy reflects the confusion and frustration on the part of professionals and women everywhere.

There are so many related issues such as osteoporosis, breast cancer, incontinence, heart disease, and more. Quite honestly, women need to be addressing these issues as early as their teens. Let me clarify say, now, that menopause is a normal, natural transition, and it is not a disease! We are so youth-oriented in this country, that most women won't even acknowledge menopause as a word. Well, I don't particularly like the word either, however, it is a reality that is better faced with information than with ignorance. In this way, you can sail through any transition, at any age, with grace, dignity, and good health!

I would like to restate that menopause is NOT a disease and don't let anyone tell you it is. Also, drugs are not the only answer, and drugs are very, very powerful substances. Taking hormones is a big deal, at any time of your life, and you should look at it that way. An even bigger concern is the predominating attitude of our society towards menopause. Menopause scares women because, as a society, we do not revere and respect mature women. Rather we idolize and revere youth and we are ever in search of it. Let us realize that we can be great at any age!

Your perception and your attitude are critical factors in any health condition or transition (such as menopause), and whether it is a positive or negative experience for you. The best thing you can do for yourself, and for all women, is to develop a new and healthy perception about yourself, your body, your health, and your choices. Reconnect to your innate feminine spirit, and know that it is a very special time in your life.

I decided to sort through the mass of information as best I could and make up my own mind about PMS, perimenopause, menopause, osteoporosis, etc. My challenge to you is to do the same thing. Read, learn, and try some of the various solutions. Remember, not everyone is the same. What works for you may not work for me or anyone else, so keep an open mind.

Many women are unaware of natural remedies and solutions for health conditions, and that may be because doctors are not aware either. Yet doctors become aware, usually through their female patients who have a positive experience with a natural solution or alternative remedy. Doctors are amazed, and then, curious. I believe it is important for each of us to learn what choices and alternatives are available, not only for ourselves, but in order to then share it with their doctors. If we don't, who will?

A number of conditions, alternatives, and remedies are mentioned in this guide and many are proven to be extremely effective. It is my belief that all symptoms, conditions, and discomforts can be alleviated *without* drugs. Even so, some of you will prefer hormone or estrogen replacement and that, indeed, is your choice, so choose it, feel good about it, and know that God has offered us many other choices in our quest for health. Again, it is important to realize that the attitude with which you approach any form of healing is significant.

Details and specifics on various pharmaceutical hormone drugs are not presented in these pages, however, you can find that information in the reference texts mentioned under "Recommended Reading." All the natural solutions and remedies in this guide are safe and encourage the body towards balance, harmony and heightened immunity. Remember, no one thing works for everyone, and everyone can and will respond differently to the same remedy.

Natural solutions and remedies take a little more time, a little more thought, and a little more effort on your part, and yet they benefit your entire body. As Plato said, *"The cure of the part should not be attempted without treatment of the whole."* A new and conscious attitude towards yourself will bring true healing into all areas of your life. Keep these directions in mind when trying something new.

Now, let me share some of what I discovered with you.

1. **Start slowly,** especially if you have never worked with alternative remedies. In time, you can and will incorporate many more. This is about changing your mind and your lifestyle to one of nurturing and choice. Make informed choices, have a little patience, and you will begin to appreciate the differences.

2. **Give things a fair chance.** If at first you don't succeed, try, try again. Doctors often prescribe several different drugs before they find the right one. Natural remedies are safe and beneficial to the entire body, so feel free to try new and various remedies.

3. **Be consistent.** Stick with something for a respectable period of time, whether it's an herb, a supplement, a diet, a relaxation or exercise program, and stay with it for few days, weeks, or months. Consistency provides best results.

4. **Be informed.** Knowledge is power. Learn all you can about your body so you can make wise choices. Relaxation and meditation are extremely helpful.,

5. **Trust your intuition and use your common sense.** Yes, you have it and so do I. Everyone has it, we just don't use it enough, so now is a good time to develop it. Your body is unique so pay close attention to it. A discomfort in your body is communicating a need. Give it some help or get some help, but in the end, trust yourself to make the best decision.

Your intentions are powerful. Intend to be better, feel better, and make wise decisions. When you are ready and willing for change, you will feel good about making your own choices. For medical advice see a doctor.

For alternative solutions or remedies, read this and continue searching and learning on your own. This information is but the tip of a great iceberg of knowledge waiting to be rediscovered and appreciated by women everywhere. Become more aware of your body and tune in to what it is telling you. When feelings of uncertainty or doubt creep in, just turn your thoughts to God and ask for help. We are all powerful, feminine spirits with great wisdom lying deep within. The wisdom of the ages and of Mother Nature is just waiting to blossom forth.

I have provided various solutions and remedies for women's symptoms. Included within those alternatives are nutrition, herbs, aromatherapy, exercise, vitamin and mineral supplements, massage, reflexology, relaxation, meditation, visualization, breathing, affirmations, plus some "home" remedies and ideas, not to mention new ways of thinking! I encourage you to try out any or all of these suggestions.

Remedies Not in this Text

It would be impossible to cover every choice, remedy, or alternative here. Even the ones discussed are in a "brief" form. Many other natural solutions, remedies, and alternatives exist which are not represented in this guide, and they can be effective too.

Solutions and remedies not mentioned include homeopathy, acupuncture, flower essences, Chinese herbs, gemstones, cleanses, chiropractic, energy work such as Reiki and healing touch, numerous other breathing techniques not described, as well as other nutritional programs and points of view. Many of these work quite well, and I have experienced a few myself. More information on other remedies can be found in various other texts, or by contacting the author of this book.

I offer you information and solutions to the standard hormone replacement therapy. It is your choice as to what to accept and what to reject. Accept my prayers and good wishes for your health, happiness, harmony, and self-empowerment no matter what you choose to do. Please enjoy the ideas presented here.

NOTE: Anything in BOLD represents, in my opinion, one of the better alternatives to try. This is based on my education, research, intuition, and are suggestions only. Everything presented is valid, yet every one may respond in a different way.

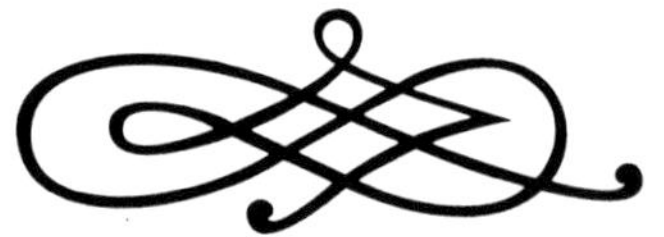

– Part I –
The Hormones

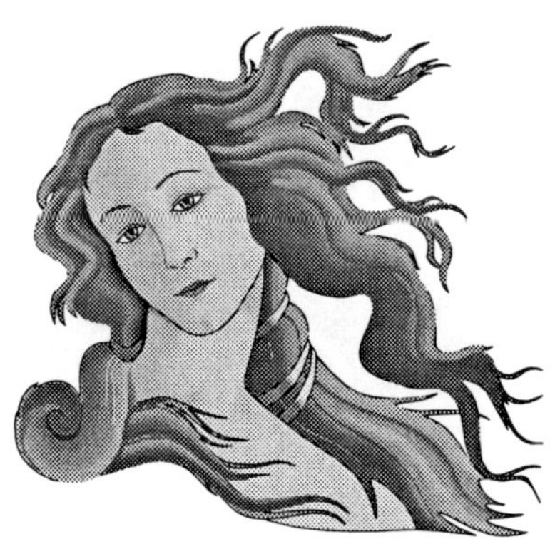

"I tried everything after my hysterectomy, and was thrilled when the natural hormones helped me feel like myself again!"

Sheri H., Age 47
Web Designer

The Hormones

Estrogen, progesterone, and testosterone are the primary sex hormones. They are affected primarily during premenopause, perimenopause, and menopause, as well as in our younger years when many experience premenstrual syndrome (PMS). First, a brief look at the reproductive or menstrual cycle that governs the production of hormones in the body which, in turn, directly affects perimenopause, pre-menopause, menopause, and PMS.

When menstruation occurs, the reproductive hormonal process begins in the brain. The hypothalamus produces a hormone called Gonadotropin-Releasing Hormone (GRH) and signals the pituitary gland which lies at the base of the brain. The pituitary gland then starts producing Follicle Stimulating Hormone (FSH) to encourage an egg in the ovary to mature, and then later sends out Luteinizing Hormone (LH) to promote ovulation. The FSH tells the ovaries to start producing several hormones including estrogen, progesterone, and androgens.

Once the ovaries start producing hormones, the pituitary stops sending out FSH. If, however, the ovaries do not respond, as may happen in perimenopause (meaning around menopause), the pituitary keeps sending out FSH, almost yelling at the ovaries to produce estrogen. This creates other responses in the brain which trigger hot flashes or other unpleasant effects. High levels of FSH indicate that you are perimenopausal. If you want to know if you are perimenopausal, ask your doctor to test your FSH level with a blood test. If your FSH level tests high, usually between 40 and 200 milli-international units per milliliter[1], this indicates you are experiencing perimenopause.

ESTROGEN is a term that refers to a class of three different estrogens that the body produces and each is a little different. They are:

ESTRADIOL — is manufactured in the ovaries and is considered the most potent form of estrogen. It is twelve times stronger than Estrone and hundreds of times stronger than estriol. Estradiol is the type of estrogen that is found in many of the hormone prescription drugs.

ESTRONE — can be manufactured from Estradiol in the liver or gut, and it is also converted from fat and muscle primarily by the adrenals.

ESTRIOL — is also manufactured in the ovaries but in a lesser quantity. This is the least potent of the estrogens and is now thought to be protective against breast cancer. This is also helpful with vaginal atrophy and dryness.

What Estrogens Do in Your Body

Besides maintaining your reproductive cycles, estrogens increase body fat, metabolize carbohydrates, affect how blood coagulates, adjusts blood pressure, assists in calcium absorption. Too much estrogen increases risk of breast and uterine cancer. These are all exceedingly important and complex biological events.

PROGESTERONE is the forgotten hormone. It is a hormone produced by the ovaries or more specifically by the corpus luteum. Everyone talks about estrogen. What isn't mentioned is progesterone and the synergistic balance between them. They work together. If you are estrogen deficient, chances are progesterone is deficient as well, and usually to a greater degree. When these two hormones are out of balance, many symptoms appear that are related to PMS, perimenopause, and menopause. Progesterone is not produced if you do not ovulate, and many women have anovulatory cycles (meaning no egg has been produced, yet you still have a menstrual peroid) as early as their thirty's. So you can be deficient in progesterone long before you're deficient in estrogen.

Progesterone prepares the endometrium for pregnancy. During pregnancy, more progesterone is produced than at any other time and may account for why pregnant women often feel so good. Natural progesterone is not found in pharmaceutical drugs. Progestins are the synthetic version of progesterone. Progestins are used in pharmaceutical drugs, such as hormone replacement prescriptions and birth control pills, and have very different effects on the body. (Please refer to section on "Hormone Replacement and Estrogen Replacement Therapy").

What Progesterone Does in Your Body

Besides playing a big role in pregnancy, progesterone also protects against fibrocystic breasts, helps use fat for energy, is a natural diuretic, antidepressant, normalizes blood clotting, facilities thyroid function, helps prevent endometrial and breast cancer, stimulates osteoblast bone building, and restores sex drive.

TESTOSTERONE is one of a class of hormones known as androgens, thought of as the male hormone, however, all women have minute amounts of testosterone which are also manufactured by the ovaries.

What Testosterone Does in Your Body

Testosterone is more predominant in males, however just like in males, testosterone affects libido as well as muscle mass, skin lubrication and also seems to play a role in preventing osteoporosis. Some signs that you may be low in testosterone are lack of libido, difficulty becoming aroused, less sensitivity in nipples and clitoris.

Fat and Adrenals Help Manufacture Estrogen

At menopause, estrogen levels decline, however, your body still produces up to forty to fifty percent of estrogen naturally from your fat cells and healthy adrenal glands. Fat plays a part in estrogen production when the ovaries slow down. Thin women may experience perimenopause and menopause a little earlier and may have more symptoms. A woman carrying a little extra fat may find perimenopause and menopause somewhat easier. However, too much fat is not healthy and is harmful to one's overall health. Making lifestyle adjustments and incorporating alternative remedies, such as diet, exercise, herbs, relaxation, and other natural remedies creates positive and beneficial effects on the way a woman feels during and after menopause.

The adrenals, located on top of the kidneys, are very much a part of the menopause or transition process. Whenever we experience stress, our adrenal glands are affected, and in our society stress is part of every day life. Often, the adrenals get worn out even before menopause! It's important to keep the adrenals strong and healthy before as well as during menopause because they play a key role in hormone production at that time. Some of the things you may notice when your adrenals get overloaded from stress are anxiety, fear, and nervousness. Relaxation, deep breathing, yoga, good diet, Vitamin C, herbs (nettles and licoric), meditation all provide nourishment and support to the adrenals.

ESTROGEN DOMINANCE or EXCESS ESTROGEN is something with which we all need to become familiar. Many conditions related to women's health are attributed to estrogen dominance, which means there is too much circulating estrogen in your system. That means even if your estrogen drops at menopause, it is still higher in comparison to progesterone. These two hormones must work together, and when one or the other is "out of sync," dramatic symptoms can result. One of the most important facts to keep in mind is that the common thread running through all women's health conditions is estrogen dominance in relationship to insufficient progesterone.[2] This brings to mind two logical questions:

(1) Why put more estrogen into a body that already has too much estrogen?

(2) Why not increase the amount of natural progesterone?

Natural progesterone (not synthetic progestin found in hormone drugs and pharmaceuticals) helps reduce and alleviate many menopausal conditions. Please see more on *natural* progesterone and its positive effects under the section "Progesterone Creams."

This is a very simple explanation of how the body produces and uses its own hormones. Most prescription hormones are not the same as the hormones produced by your body and, therefore, produce side effects. Some women cannot tolerate prescription hormones for many reasons, perhaps because they are artificially manufactured in a laboratory and their body is too sensitive. Prescription drugs sold under a trade name and patent are not natural, they are synthetic (manufactured) products. Natural products, foods, herbs, etc. cannot be patented and, therefore, are not usually "prescribed" or recommended by doctors, partly because doctors are not aware of them or educated about them.

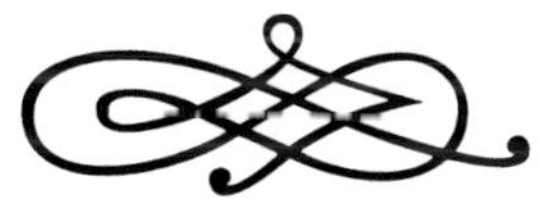

Menopause

Menopause a new beginning! Yes, really. It is also a normal and natural transition. Unfortunately, most women dread the word "menopause" and worry that life is over. We think of menopause as a loss of our femininity or sexuality and diminishing attractiveness to men. This is a distressing myth that our culture has encouraged, and it is time for a change! In many cultures, mature women are revered and respected. We need to develop more of that kind of perception! Guess what? It starts with you and me.

Menopause does not need to be traumatic. In fact, it truly is a normal and natural transition. It is an awakening of spirit, and as Margaret Mead said ***"The most creative force in the world is a menopausal woman with zest!"*** As our body adjusts to the hormonal changes taking place, so does our spirit adjust and open to greater insights and wisdom from within.

In puberty, we *expected* to make a transition as our bodies developed and hormones went wild. So now, we must expect and allow menopause to transition us to a deeper awareness of ourselves as we become the wise women that we truly are. Menopause, just like at puberty, concerns hormones adjusting and balancing themselves either up or down. This affects us physically, mentally, emotionally, and spiritually.

Menopause defined is the normal, natural transition a woman experiences as she ends her reproductive years. In spite of what you may have heard, menopause is NOT a disease. It is the cessation of estrogen production from the ovaries, and the complete termination of menses for up to one full year. The average age for this to occur is around age fifty, but may occur as early as age thirty-five or as late as age fifty-five. Several factors can contribute to early or premature menopause and they are:

> **Surgical removal of ovaries, genetics, smoking, poor diet, severe infections, lack of exercise or obsessive exercising, ovarian infections, chemotherapy.**

The unpleasant effects of menopause are what we are concerned about, and there is valid reason to believe our American lifestyle is a culprit. What's interesting is that in Asia, they don't even have a word for PMS, menopause, or hot flashes! These menopausal symptoms will be addressed in "Part II."

Other symptoms of menopause include:

> **Hot flashes, warm flashes, irregular periods, fibroids, fatigue, heart palpitations, minor depression, headaches, migraines, acne, mood swings, anxiety attacks, lack of concentration, decreased libido, fibrocystic breasts, sleep disorders, weight gain, fatigue, urinary infections, incontinence, vaginal dryness or atrophy, digestive problems, skin and hair changes.**

As one of many women entering an exciting and transformative time of life, you can be one of the first to bring a new image and perception to menopause. Whether you know it or not, YOU ARE IN CHARGE and YOU DO HAVE CHOICES! We women are an influential force and have a powerful voice. Let us be heard.

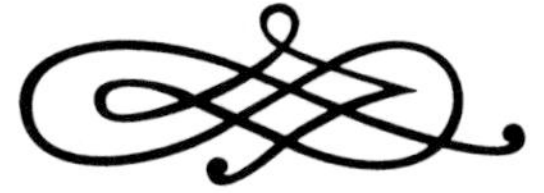

Perimenopause
A.K.A. Premenopause

Perimenopause means "around" menopause. Often times, once you makes it through perimenopause, the rest is a breeze. What most of us don't realize is that many hormonal problems or imbalances experienced at age thirty-five and into our early forty's are related to premenopause or perimenopause. For example, PMS, menstrual headaches, and sore breasts fall within perimenopausal symptoms, and I, too, have experienced this. You too may be experiencing these kinds of symptoms and not realize their significance. So what is perimenopause?

Perimenopause is also known as pre-menopause, and it is the period of time between the normal reproductive cycle and menopause. Perimenopause also incorporates the time just following menopause as well. Basically, it is a time when hormones begin to fluctuate and create imbalances in the body which, in turn, create unpleasant symptoms.

Symptoms of perimenopause can begin as early as age thirty! What are they? Perimenopausal symptoms are related to menopausal symptoms, and both are about imbalanced hormones). It's just a matter of which ones and their intensity. If you have symptoms not specifically mentioned here, they are still real and valid and simply reinforce the uniqueness of you. No two women are alike, and no two women will experience menopause exactly alike either.

The changes we experience in and through our body at perimenopause and menopause provide us with many opportunities to make other changes in our life. It is unfortunate to have to say that our modern, technological American lifestyle is a contributing factor to the unpleasant symptoms of perimenopause and menopause as well as our perception of it. Yet, it is within our power to make positive and healthy choices for ourselves and to create a new perception of the menopausal woman in America as a wise woman.

I encourage you to take steps, no matter how small, towards making significant changes in your life. Small steps are easier to incorporate than giant leaps. Learn which alternatives appeal to you whether it be nutrition, exercise, supplements, herbs, or even prescription hormones. You have a choice! At the least, make an informed choice, and then start slow and easy.

Again, perimenopause is the beginning of a dynamic transition. So pay attention early. Changes in your physical body brings changes in your attitude and ideas. Take advantage of this opportunity to grow and respond to life in new and exciting ways. Be creative. Take up new forms of expression that reveal the inner beauty and wisdom awakening within you.

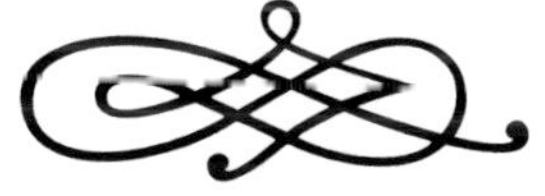

Hormone Replacement and Estrogen Replacement Therapy

Hormone or Estrogen Replacement Therapy are the common responses to perimenopause and menopause by most doctors. Yet there are still many unanswered questions about its long term safety, as well as some already known problems with these therapies.

Hormone Replacement Therapy (HRT) and Estrogen Replacement Therapy (ERT) are two approaches physicians use to replace hormones in women during menopause. The difference is this: HRT uses a combination of estrogen and progestin while ERT uses only estrogen. The hormones used is both instances, for the most part, are not natural hormones nor are they identical to the human body's hormones. They are manufactured or manipulated in a lab so that a company can "patent" them for sale. Premarin, for example, once the most prescribed drug in America (I believe it is now Viagra), is derived from pregnant mare's urine.

Most times when HRT or ERT are prescribed, a pre-formulated drug is given. So, you receive the same prescription as your neighbor down the street. As you must know, you are unique, special, and different from your neighbor. Therefore, the type and amount of each hormone you need may be different too. Have your hormone levels checked in advance of taking a prescription, and be aware that hormone levels fluctuate, not only from woman to woman, but from day to day! Checking you hormone levels several times throughout a month is a good idea. If you choose HRT or ERT, you can now request natural hormones, however, they need to be made at a compounding pharmacy.

A compounding pharmacy is equipped to make up (compound) the appropriate levels of each hormone especially for your body from *natural substances* (from soy or wild yam) with a doctor's prescription. If you decide to use hormones to assist you through menopause, this is your best choice. This requires finding a physician who is willing and knows how to write this kind of prescription.

Significant Reasons to Take HRT

There are some claims that HRT prevents osteoporosis and heart disease, however, recent studies coming out are disproving this. Using HRT or ERT on a short term basis may be a viable alternative to help reduce severe hot flashes or vaginal dryness. "Short term" being defined as several months to a year. Most women are free of hot flashes within two years or less, and vaginal dryness can be remedied with creams and herbs.

If you have additional concerns in these areas, please refer to the sections on "Heart Disease" and "Osteoporosis." Also, begin to educate yourself. There are significant, negative side effects to ERT which you will want to know about, and if breast or uterine cancer runs in your family, ERT is definitely not your best choice.

ERT Increases Risk of:

- Breast cancer
- Growth of fibroids
- Blood clots or breast fibroids in women with a history of these conditions
- Uterine cancer
- Gallbladder and liver problems

HRT also comes with its own bag of side effects.

Possible HRT Side Effects:

- Increased risk of heart disease or stroke (due to the progestin).
- Artificially manipulates the natural menstrual cycle and may cause menstrual bleeding even after menopause.
- Difficult to find combination and dosage to effectively relieve symptoms.

Other Complaints Associated With ERT and HRT:

- Bloating
- Irregular bleeding
- Headaches
- Hair loss
- Elevated blood pressure
- Yeast infections
- Nausea
- Emotional imbalance
- Abdominal cramps
- Weight gain
- Breast tenderness
- Depression

One of the most important facts to note is that too much estrogen contributes to all menopausal conditions. Rather than taking more estrogen, why not add natural progesterone to balance out this discrepancy. **NATURAL PROGESTERONE** duplicates the body's progesterone exactly and is shown to be extremely effective for many conditions. Progesterone is a sex hormone with at least as much importance as estrogen, but it has been given far less attention. Please refer to section on "Progesterone Creams" for more explanation and information on this subject.

PROGESTIN is the synthetic form of progesterone found in combination with estrogen in many of the HRT prescription drugs and in birth control pills. Progestin and progesterone are often used interchangeably, but they are very different. Progestin causes many adverse side effects of its own.

Possible Adverse Side Effects of Progestin:

- Diminishes positive effects of estrogens on cardiovascular system
- May increase breast cancer risk
- May cause acne
- May cause breakthrough bleeding or change in menses
- Sodium and fluid retention which leads to hypertension
- Depression, nausea, insomnia, headaches
- Increase or decrease in weight
- May decrease glucose tolerance (diabetic patients must be carefully monitored)

If you do decide to use estrogen or estrogen/progestin, there are several ways to take these drugs. They come in pills to be taken orally, patches which deliver the hormone through the skin, and creams or gels which also deliver hormones through the skin. Oral prescriptions come in various strengths, and all drugs taken orally must pass through the liver. On the other hand, patches allow the hormones to be delivered directly into the bloodstream through the skin. Most hormones that come in patches are natural, that is, they are derived from natural sources such as soy products or wild yam. Creams and gels are also absorbed through the skin or through the sensitive vaginal tissues and bypass the liver.

Although this is an extremely important and extensive topic, this guide does not examine all the various prescription hormone drugs. Remember that prescription hormones include not only Premarin, Prempro, Provera, but many others including all birth control pills which also contain synthetic hormones.

It is my belief that, in most situations, all symptoms and concerns can be addressed through natural alternatives. If interested, you can easily find more information on this topic. See the "Recommended Reading List" at the end of this book.

Deciding To Stop ERT or HRT

Once you start taking ERT or HRT, can you stop? Yes. However, if you decide to stop taking estrogen or hormone replacement, do so slowly over a period of time. Take a month, two months, or up to six months, if needed and if you are not going to a natural hormone treatment. If you stop "cold turkey" you are likely to experience withdrawal symptoms. It is important to do this gently because it allows your body to adjust more easily. You can start tapering off the pills in several different ways, and you may wish to consult with your physician or a holistic practitioner for some guidance. One way is to start alternating dosages or skipping days between pills. Have a plan and follow it. Then, pay attention to your body. Your body is very wise, and it will let you know what it needs.

In addition, feel free to include alternative remedies such as herbs, vitamins, exercise, dietary changes. These can be started concurrently without a problem.

On the other hand, with the assistance of a health practitioner, you can also get natural hormone products to replace the drugs, and they can be used as soon as you stop the HRT or ERT. This needs professional guidance and can be done by immediately stopping the synthetic hormones and replacing them with natural hormones. Please consult someone who is knowledgeable in this area.

Hormone Balance

We cannot underestimate the power of hormones in the body. The value and importance of estrogen and, particularly, progesterone, affects every woman. Our culture and health care industry are so enamored with estrogen, it stands to reason that progesterone is often overlooked. This is incredible, since nearly all women's conditions are based on balancing hormones, and that includes estrogen *and* progesterone. Therefore, it is essential to keep both hormones in balance, and when they are not in balance, a hormone imbalance exists.

What is hormone imbalance? Hormone imbalance is when estrogen and/or progesterone are not in balance with each other. Hormone imbalance is related to all women's conditions, and even some men's conditions. The primary hormones for women are estrogen and progesterone, with a small amount of testosterone (important, but not as significant as progesterone). Be aware, there are at least three different estrogens, and they are not all equal in their effect on the body (see section on "Hormones"). Our industrialized lifestyle affects the hormones mostly by increasing estrogen, or estrogen-like compounds, and reducing progesterone. Women can end up with too much estrogen, and this is called Estrogen Dominance or Excess Estrogen. How does this happen? What increases estrogen in the body? Some things that increase estrogen are:

- American Industrialized Lifestyle in General
- Poor Nutrition (including fast foods, processed foods, hydrogenated oils, and more)
- Red Meat and Dairy Products (coming from estrogen-fed beef and poultry)
- Lack of Exercise
- Alcohol
- Drugs (legal or not)
- Xenoestrogens (primarily Petrochemicals which come from plastics, pesticides, household cleaners, etc.)

A word on xenoestrogens, which means "foreign" estrogens. When these products enter the body through skin, nose, mouth, they act like estrogen and connect to the same receptors as estrogen does. Xenoestrogens are very powerful and toxic. Since there is no way to totally eliminate these chemicals from our life, it is important for us to limit exposure to them whenever possible. That means chemical glues, dyes, gasoline products, exhaust from cars, toxic and poisonous household cleaners, plastics, and much more. Perhaps this is as good a reason as any to use natural and/or organic products and cleaners. Many people develop allergies to some of these products. That is a sign that your body may be overloaded or cannot tolerate them anymore.

As for estrogen, be aware that, in most cases, you do not need additional estrogen. Not only can too much estrogen (especially estradiol and estrone) increase your risk of breast and uterine cancer, estrogen helps to increase and retain weight. Women, I know, want to lose weight, not put more on. Though weight is not the most dangerous side-effect of estrogen, it is one women can relate to easily. See the list of negative effects cited in the section on "Hormone Replacement and Estrogen Replacement Therapy" to find out more about what too much estrogen can do.

Knowing there are three different estrogens, let's look at the form of estrogen called estriol. Estriol is, by far, the safest form of estrogen. It is very effective for vaginal conditions, especially for vaginal atrophy and dry vagina. In addition, studies are finding that estriol can actually be protective against breast and uterine cancer, whereas estradiol and estrone contribute to or aggravate cancer. Most pharmaceutical estrogens are estradiol.

A good word on progesterone. This is, in my opinion, the happy hormone. When women are pregnant, progesterone begins to increase and becomes the primary hormone at the time of birth. A woman's normal production of progesterone is approximately twenty to twenty-four milligrams of progesterone a day. A pregnant woman in the third trimester, is manufacturing approximately four hundred milligrams per day! Once a woman gives birth, her progesterone level drops instantly and dramatically. When I discovered this, I wondered why the medical profession did not connect postpartum depression with this fact, and indeed, it is related.

The women's conditions mentioned in this book and many others, are affected by a drop or lack of progesterone, and at times, estrogen. Since progesterone is the biological precursor to estrogen, it is critical to have progesterone. Many times, adding progesterone alone can alleviate some estrogen related conditions such as hot flashes or dry vagina. Progesterone is safe and effective. That is only true if you are using natural progesterone. As discussed in the section "Hormone Replacement and Estrogen Replacement Therapy," please do not confuse synthetic Progestin with natural progesterone. A fact often misstated by doctors as well. You must know the difference and ask! Progestin has many unpleasant side effects, while progesterone helps with almost every female condition.

Essentially, the balance of hormones needs to be looked at carefully by you and your doctor. If a woman has too much estrogen, as they often do, it seems illogical to prescribe more estrogen in the form of estrogen or hormone replacement therapy. If a woman is having trouble with ovulation, it seems logical to add progesterone instead of estrogen. It is ovulation that creates the corpus luteum where progesterone is manufactured. Thus, if there is no ovulation, then no progesterone is made. Progesterone is also important in retaining and growing a baby. A client once told me she had seven miscarriages. It was only on her last one that her doctor recommended progesterone suppositories! She carried that child to full term.

Please, please watch and adjust your lifestyle in order to begin bringing your body and hormones back into balance! Avoid xenoestrogens and petrochemicals as much as possible. Take a close look at the Checklist For Estrogen Dominance and be aware if you are experiencing any of the symptoms from headaches to thyroid problems to hypoglycemia (low blood sugar). Be concerned and careful about what you eat, drink, and smell. Your body is your temple. You are not an island. You and I are significant players in a world that needs more care, understanding, communication, health, and peace. Start with yourself and start now.

Checklist For Estrogen Dominance

How do you know if you have too much estrogen? Here is a checklist which may be helpful to you. This list of symptoms reflect estrogen dominance according to Dr. John R. Lee.[3] Read through them, and mark the ones that apply to you. Use the following numbers to help rate your symptoms.

0 = no symptoms;
1 = mild, occasional symptoms;
2 = moderate, noticeable but not debilitating;
3 = severe, interferes with normal routine, debilitating

Allergies .... ________
Breast Tenderness .... ________
Decreased Libido .... ________
Minor Depression .... ________
Fatigue .... ________
Fibrocystic Breasts .... ________
Fibroids, Uterine .... ________
Foggy Thinking .... ________
Headaches .... ________
Hypoglycemia .... ________
Increased Blood Clotting .... ________
Infertility .... ________
Irritability .... ________
Memory Loss .... ________
Osteoporosis .... ________
Premenopausal Bone Loss .... ________
PMS .... ________
Thyroid Dysfunction .... ________
Uterine Cancer .... ________
Water Retention and Bloating .... ________
Weight Gain, esp. around abdomen,
hips and thighs .... ________
Gallbladder Disease .... ________
Autoimmune Disorders .... ________
Acceleration of Aging Process/Wrinkles ... ________

Total ________

This is a way to become more aware of your symptoms and determine if they might be related to your perimenopausal or menopausal situation. The higher your score, the more excess estrogen. If you are concerned, get a saliva test to check your hormone levels.

1. Sandra Cabot, M.D., *Smart Medicine for Menopause, Hormone Replacement Therapy and its Natural Alternatives*, Avery Publishing Group, New York, 1995.

2. John R. Lee, M.D., *What Your Doctor May Not Tell You About Menopause*, Warner Books, New York, 1996.

3. John R. Lee, M.D., *What Your Doctor May Not Tell You About Menopause*, Warner Books, New York, 1996, pg. 42.

– Part II –
Conditions

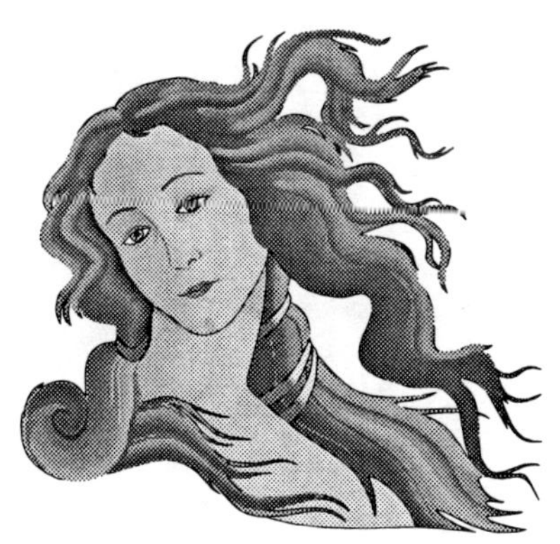

"Finally! A book that gives some quick and effective solutions, and I don't have to read ten others."

Laura J., Age 49,
Executive Director, Health Center

Bladder

Bladder problems include incontinence, infections, and cystitis. These conditions affect many women during perimenopause and menopause. As you approach menopause, it is not uncommon for the bladder muscles to weaken, lose elasticity, for infections to occur, or to experience incontinence.

Incontinence of the bladder is one of the worst feelings you can experience, yet this is not uncommon just before or after menopause. Incontinence is when you lose tone in and around the bladder muscles. Stress incontinence is when things as simple as laughing, coughing, or sneezing cause urine leakage. Exercise and other normal activities may put stress on the bladder too. There is also urge incontinence which refers to urine leakage that occurs as soon as the urge to void is felt. In this case, never wait to relieve your bladder.

Several factors contribute to incontinence including pregnancies, abdominal surgeries, medications, alcohol, infections, and more. Emotional and/or physical stress and lack of exercise are also contributing factors. During menopause, the walls of the bladder become thinner and have less elasticity due to the hormonal changes in the body. However, you can improve those muscles and bring back good tone. One of the best ways is by doing **Kegel exercises.**

Bladder infections are also be a problem. Cystitis and bladder infections cause painful and frequent urination. The urge to urinate continues even after you've emptied your bladder. If you notice blood in the urine, this indicates a serious problem so do not hesitate to contact your doctor. Generally, your body gives you signals at the beginning of an infection such as pressure or tingling. Precaution and early detection before things get worse are the best remedies.

If you think you have a bladder infection, you can purchase a product called Dipstick from the drugstore. The tip of the strip changes color when dipped in urine and indicates the presence of bacteria. Be sure to follow the directions on the package to obtain accurate results. If in doubt or in pain, contact a health care professional.

The usual prescription for infections and cystitis is antibiotics. Whenever you take antibiotics, be aware that as the "bad" bacteria is being killed off, so is the "friendly" bacteria or flora that your intestines need. It's a good idea to take a reliable form of acidophilus during and after the antibiotic treatment in order to replenish the "friendly" flora that are destroyed. Your body will thank you.

ALTERNATIVE CHOICES

- Nutrition – Vitamins – Minerals
- Tips on Emptying Bladder
- Aromatherapy
- Herbs
- Kegel Exercises
- Affirmations

Nutrition - Vitamins – Minerals

Most women who have had cystitis or bladder infections are aware of that standby remedy cranberry juice. You may also include green drinks (like chlorophyll) and green foods (leafy greens). Eliminate caffeine, coffee, colas, chocolate, and mucus forming foods such as dairy. Other suggestions:

- **Drink lots of cranberry juice (sugarless, if possible) and water throughout the day**
- Vitamin C – 4,000 to 5,000 mg daily divided in doses
- Acidophilus – 2 to 3 times a day
(Buttermilk is also good to drink)
- Calcium and Magnesium, in balance, is helpful

Tips On Emptying Bladder

- Completely void each time you urinate. A way to accomplish this is to press down behind your pubic bone with your fingertips or hand.
- Don't wait when you have to urinate. At the first sensation of the urge find restroom, whether at home, at work or shopping. Holding it in only irritates the bladder more.
- Urinate after intercourse to prevent bacteria from backing up into the bladder.

Herbs

Echinacea/Goldenseal, Cranberry, Cranberry Buchu (NSP Brand), Juniper Berries, Alfalfa, **Cornsilk,** Garlic, Parsley, Slippery Elm, Uva Ursi

Aromatherapy

Lavender, Juniper, Cedarwood, Sandalwood

Sitz Baths

Soaking in a warm, bubbly bath is wonderful for the entire body, mind, and spirit. A Sitz bath is directed to the perineum area around the urethra and is soothing, healing and relaxing. If desired, add four to six drops of an Essential Oil to the Sitz bath or a bubble bath. Rest and soak for about twenty minutes.

Kegel Exercises

Kegel exercises are used for bladder control and pelvic strengthening. They strengthen the muscles around your vagina and urinary opening that help to support the uterus, bladder, and rectum. Some exercises can be done anywhere, anytime, for example sitting in your car, waiting in line, or standing at the kitchen sink. You will notice a marked improvement in your muscles after a week or two, and then continue doing the exercises regularly.

- In order to find the correct muscles, contract your vaginal muscles to stop the flow of urine while urinating. Hold it for as long as you can before releasing the flow.
- To improve bladder control, again contract your vaginal muscles while urinating. Begin by pushing the urine flow out strongly, then decreasing the flow until hardly any flow appears. Repeat this process until your bladder is empty.
- Contract your vaginal muscles (as if stopping the flow of urine) and hold for the count of five, then release for a count of five. Repeat this sequence up to ten times, and do it a minimum of five times a day. This can be done anywhere without anyone knowing.

- Contract and release your vaginal muscles in rapid successions for a sequence of thirty. Repeat this exercise five to ten times a day.
- Once your muscles are toned, you can do these exercises once a day to keep them in shape.
- To obtain quicker results and add resistance to your exercises, try the Kegel Exerciser® (see "Resources" section). This is a device which allows you to strengthen the pelvic floor muscles in order to prevent incontinence and leakage.

AFFIRMATIONS

I am in control of my life.

I release the old and welcome everything new into my life.

It is safe for me to express my emotions.

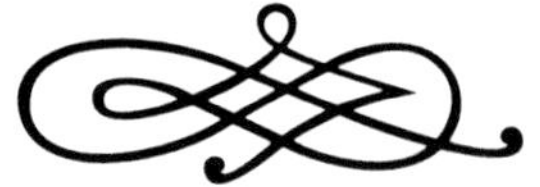

Breast Cancer

One in three people will get cancer in their lifetime according to statistics, and one in nine women will get breast cancer. Breast cancer is one of the predominant fears for every woman, no matter what her age.

Excess estrogen or estrogen dominance has been associated with cancer in women. The biggest choice you will ever make at menopause is whether or not to use estrogen replacement therapy (ERT). The "implied" benefits of ERT are reduced risk of heart disease and protection from osteoporosis. This is being researched and may not be true at all. The truth is that the jury is not in on this subject, and there are other choices! Please read the sections on "Heart Disease" and "Osteoporosis" for more discussion on these issues.

A love affair with estrogen has been playing out since the 60's. Believing it is the source of youth, femininity, and perennial sexual attractiveness and desire, women and women's doctors have not yet asked enough questions about its safety or its risks. Research is just beginning to look at the long term effects of ERT and its affect on breast cancer among other things.

Most studies indicate there is greater risk of developing uterine and/or breast cancer if you are taking unopposed estrogen (estrogen alone). Estrogen is found in all birth control pills, Premarin (which is one of the largest selling drugs in the U.S.), and other drugs prescribed at menopause. Some pharmaceutical drugs prescribed at menopause now contain both estrogen and progestin, which is the synthetic form of progesterone, and unfortunately, both have their unpleasant side effects (See section on "Hormone Replacement and Estrogen Replacement Therapy").

Unlike fibrocystic breasts, a cancerous lump found in the breast does not move freely, is not tender, does not fluctuate in size, and does not go away.

Other factors believed to contribute to breast cancer include:

- High animal fat diet
- Stress
- Smoking – contributory factor in all cancers

- High sugar consumption
- Alcohol
- Lower selenium level
- Environmental toxins

ALTERNATIVE CHOICES

- Nutrition - Vitamins – Minerals
- Aromatherapy
- Herbs
- Visualization
- Affirmations

Nutrition – Vitamins – Minerals

The food you eat has a tremendous effect or your health and immunity. There are many alternatives in this area and, again, you need to make a choice for one that appeals to you. Here's a couple to consider:

- **Macrobiotic diet** which include lots of sea vegetables, lightly steamed foods, grains, and elimination of most popular fat and fast food items. This is a very precise diet, so check your library or bookstore for books on this program, or look for practitioners of macrobiotics in your area.
- A raw foods and juice fast encourages elimination and detoxification. The Optimum Health Institute located in Lemon Grove, California, specializes in raw foods and juices. Many people with health challenges, including cancer, visit this Institute and experience surprisingly positive results.
- **Periodic juice or vegetable fasts** can be helpful in preventing cancer. You too can prepare a mini-fresh, raw fruit or vegetable fast/diet for a day or several days. Check your library or bookstore for more information and books on this topic.
- Get books on nutrition and cancer; one is *Beating Cancer With Nutrition* by Dr. Patrick Quillin.

Other important guidelines to follow include:

- Reduce animal fats
- **Eliminate alcohol completely**
- Take antioxidants (Vitamins A, C, E, Selenium)

- Vitamin C with Bioflavanoids
- Cruciferous vegetables – broccoli, cabbage, Brussels sprouts, kale, etc.
- Reduce or eliminate processed sugars
- Eat soy based foods – tofu, miso, etc.
- Take beta carotene
- Increase Acidophilus intake
- Eat high fiber foods – dietary fiber increases fecal excretion of estrogen and other toxins

Herbs

Red Clover, Echinacea, Goldenseal, Pau D'Arco, **Shark Cartilage,** Burdock

Essiac Tea – Native American herbal recipe made famous in 1920's and available in most health food stores

Green Tea – known for its anti-carcinogenic and anti-tumor effects

Aromatherapy

Rose, Cypress, Eucalyptus, Geranium, Lavender, Lemon, Tea Tree

Visualization

Relax. Take several slow, deep breaths and imagine your immune system gaining strength with each breath. Then picture, imagine or just believe your body eliminating the cancer cells, just like Pac men gobbling them up. Put your loving attention on the area needing healing and do this three or four times a day for at least thirty minutes or longer.

AFFIRMATIONS

I lovingly release all past hurts.

I am renewed with every breath.

I am free to express the real me.

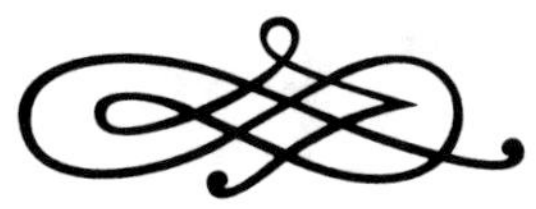

Constipation

Constipation is more common than you might imagine and not only among women at menopause. However, it is a typical problem whenever the hormones start to shift and change. Many women experience constipation the week or so prior to starting their periods. Often considered another PMS symptom, it can become even more of a concern during the menopause years.

So, what is constipation? Constipation according to Dorland's *Medical Dictionary* is "infrequent or difficult evacuation of the feces." It is also anything other than regular, easy, well-formed bowel movements. Our bodies were designed to evacuate waste products after taking in a meal. If that is so, then three meals a day means three bowel movements a day! How many of us are that lucky? Many people are lucky to have one bowel movement a day. The sad fact is that it is not unusual for people to go several days without having a bowel movement. This is very unhealthy and can even be dangerous.

Keeping the colon and elimination channels clear and flowing are essential to good health, not only during menopause but throughout your life. It is believed that ninety percent of all disease starts in the colon. The reason it is so important at menopause is that the colon also helps eliminate excess estrogen from the system. If that does not happen, estrogen stays in your system and can actually be reabsorbed. It may be of interest to know that other conditions such as, sinus problems, low back pains, or headaches can be triggered by a toxic colon as well.

A number of things that contribute to constipation include:

- Lack of bulk in diet
- Lack of moisture
- Lack of movement or exercise
- White flour, sugar, meat, alcohol, cheese – all slow down the digestive tract
- Iron supplements – which can cause other digestive distresses as well

- Not moving your bowels upon the initial "urge" to do so. So, don't wait!
- Stress
- Aspirin
- Birth Control Pills
- Cortisone Drugs
- Antibiotics, which totally disrupts good flora in the colon

Constipation may be resolved in a number of natural ways. You may even have your favorite! First, it is a good idea to determine if you are chronically constipated or if it's a recent problem. For example, recent problems occurring from hospital food, laying in bed, and no exercise are guaranteed to stop you up. This type of problem can usually be resolved by getting back to your normal routine (as long as you are not constipated to begin with).

Chronic constipation means you may have been that way most of your life or for at least a significant time period. This is not unusual. If it's a chronic condition, it may take a little more time and a little more effort to retrain your colon muscles. There is always some stress or emotional situation that accompanies chronic constipation.

Enemas and colonics are for emergencies only! Sometimes they can be utilized for a "cleansing" program. However, they do not resolve the problem. Remember, the goal is to have regular, well-formed daily bowel movements.

Psyllium seeds and powder are not highly recommended, because they can be even more constipating especially for women. A better solution would be a sugar-free soluble fiber that is derived from guar gum, called Benefiber® (see "Resources").

The best solution includes a combination of lifestyle adjustments, including improved nutrition, added fiber to diet, exercise, and supplements or herbs, all of which are safe, healthy and long lasting.

ALTERNATIVE CHOICES

- Nutrition
- Herbs
- Exercise
- Affirmations

Nutrition

Helpful guidelines for everyone:

1. Eat more foods with **fiber.** Fiber improves transit time through the colon and helps the stool to form. Fiber absorbs waste and moves it out.

   Foods with the highest fiber content are in the following order:

   - Unprocessed whole grains (rice, wheat, corn, barley, rye, oats, millet, etc)
   - Legumes (peas, beans, lentils, nuts, seeds, dried fruit)
   - Root Vegetables (carrots, yams, beets, turnips and parsnips)
   - Fruit and Leafy Greens including lettuce, cabbage and celery
   - NO FIBER is found in meat, dairy, cheese, fish, chicken, processed foods, sweets, etc.

2. Chew foods thoroughly to mix with saliva and begin digestion in the mouth.

3. **Eat prunes, prune juice, figs.**

4. Add more moisture and bulk to colon (for dry stools). Include:

   - Aloe Vera Juice
   - Pine Nuts
   - Slippery Elm Powder
   - Seaweed and Sea Vegetables
   - Flax Seeds

5. Acidophilus – use enteric-coated capsules or yogurt (unflavored, full fat, or low fat). Excellent for colon and aids in digestive disturbances as well.

Herbs

Cascara Sagrada – Helps paristalsis of muscles, use cautiously and start slowly

Senna – Can be harsh, yet works, so use in moderation

Dandelion – Helps with gas and other digestive woes

Betonite Clay – Liquid or powder pulls out toxins

Glycerine Suppositories – helps move bowels quickly

Benefiber® – Natural vegetable soluble fiber

TEAS: Senna, Chamomile

Exercise

- Get up and move, especially if you sit at a desk all day!
- **Movement** of a any kind stimulates and works the muscles of the colon.
- Walking, Rebounding on a Mini-Trampoline, Swimming, etc.
- All Sports are Great
- Yoga Helps Tone All Muscles
- Yoga Stomach Lifts

AFFIRMATIONS

I release, I let go and I allow life to flow.

As I release old patterns, joy fills my life.

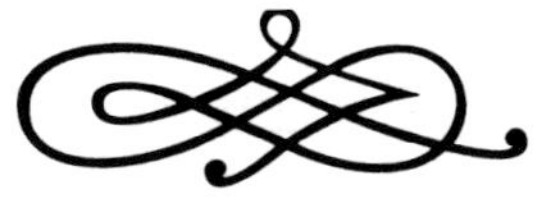

Endometriosis

Endometriosis is unique to the twentieth century. It is a condition where the endometrial cells, which grow inside the uterus, grow elsewhere. During the menstrual cycle, the endometrium builds up with blood, preparing for eventual conception. If that does not happen, the cells are then sloughed off during the process of menstruation. Endometriosis means that these cells have grown outside the uterus where they do not belong, such as the fallopian tubes, in or on the ovaries, on the outer surface of the uterus and other pelvic organs such as the colon or the bladder. When this happens, the cells cause the various pelvic organs to bind together.

These endometrial cells are affected by the hormones during the menstrual cycle. They increase in size and swell up with blood, just as the cells do inside the uterus. Then, they bleed into the surrounding tissues. This bleeding, no matter how small, causes inflammation and adhesions, which can be very painful. The adhesions created are not easy to diagnose. Often, they are not large enough to show on an X-ray or sonogram. Laproscopy (a minimally invasive surgery allowing a doctor to view inside the abdomen with a small scope) can be helpful in this regard.

The symptoms associated with endometriosis include incapacitating pain in the uterus, lower back, the organs in the pelvic cavity prior to and during menstruation, intermittent pain through the menstrual cycle, excessive bleeding including passing of large clots during menses, painful intercourse; nausea, vomiting, constipation during menses, and infertility. Because menstruation is heavy, iron deficiency anemia is common.[1]

The cause of endometriosis is not clear. Some argue that it's "retrograde" menstruation where cells are forced back up through the fallopian tubes. Others suggest a possible embryonic defect during fetus development. Unidentified as yet, the cause may be related to the sensitivity of the embryo to our modern petrochemical compounds (plastics, pesticides, etc.) with potent estrogen-like activity and considered highly toxic.

In any case, it is a twentieth century problem, once termed the "working woman's disease." Traditional medical treatments are generally not very successful.

Some traditional medical treatments include creating a false pregnancy by using large doses of progestins over a long period of time, or surgically removing the lesions. The most drastic approach is hysterectomy. These have not proved to be very successful, and can even create more problems. A piece of good news is that menopause is a cure! However,do not wait for that!

ALTERNATIVE CHOICES

- Nutrition
- Progesterone Cream
- Herbs
- Aromatherapy
- Visualization
- Affirmations

Nutrition

- **Iron – use Floradex, liquid herbal iron tonic**
- **Cut back on caffeine, sugar, and alcoholic beverages**
- Eat iron enriched foods such as molasses, eggs, liver, meat, whole grains, green leafy vegetables, almonds, avocados, beets.
- Take a multiple vitamin/mineral supplement
- B Complex Vitamins
- Vitamin C with Bioflavanoids 1000 to 3000 mg/day

Progesterone

Dr. John Lee suggests **using Progesterone Cream** which blocks further proliferation of endometrial cells. Use natural progesterone cream from day six to day twenty-six of the cycle each month. Use one ounce of cream, per week, for three weeks, stopping just before the expected period. This treatment requires patience. Over four to six months, the monthly pains gradually subside.

Herbs

Red Raspberry – relaxes, strengthens, and nourishes uterus

Siberian Ginseng – helps normalize body processes, also provides energy

Aromatherapy

Geranium – balances hormones

Clary Sage – balances and helps with cramps

Visualization

Visualization encourages significant changes at the cellular level. As you breathe and relax, close your eyes and imagine the lesions healing and disappearing. I often use my Guardian Angel and a spiritual vacuum cleaner to assist in removing all the dark spots and old blood. Then imagine applying a healing cream to any and all areas needing it.

AFFIRMATIONS

My female organs are healthy throughout.

My body and hormones are perfectly balanced.

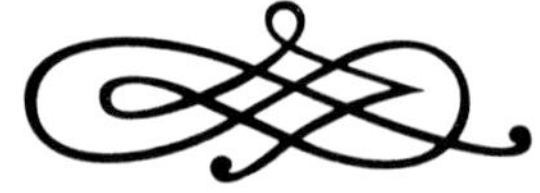

Fibrocystic Breasts

Sore breasts, known as fibrocystic breasts, are a pervasive problem. Fully, fifty to seventy-five percent of women have fibrocystic breasts.[2] This condition can cause minor discomfort or it can be extremely debilitating so that even walking brings extreme pain. Take heart, you are not alone, and there is help. I can't help but think that perceiving and accepting our bodies and femininity as beautiful expressions of life would be a first and necessary step towards health.

Fibrocystic breasts are benign breast lumps that feel tender, move freely under the skin and often fluctuate with your menstrual cycle. The breast is an estrogen sensitive area and if there is too much estrogen circulating in your system, you experience uncomfortable effects. Fewer cysts seem to form after menopause, so this problem appears to be more prevalent during perimenopause or during regular reproductive cycles.

Let's look at fibrocystic breast disease as it is called. First, it is not a disease! Rather it is a condition related to our dietary and environmental lifestyle. Second, be assured that the literature states breast pain is not an indication of cancer nor an indication of increased risk for breast cancer. However, what does appear to contribute to fibrocystic breasts, as well as breast cancer, is a high fat or high caffeine diet.

Contributing factors include:

- Caffeine – coffee, teas and chocolate and over-the-counter medications of which many contain caffeine including aspirin
- High Fat Diet – without enough fiber and antioxidants
- Excess Estrogen – either from foods, drugs, irregular menstrual cycles, or Estrogen Replacement Therapy

Fibrocystic breast problems respond quite well to natural remedies. Natural therapies such as diet, exercise, massage, herbs, etc. are very helpful. If this is one of your concerns, try one or more of the following alternatives. Remember, as with any condition, you may need to try several things before you find just the right one or combination that works best for you. The first thing to try, in my opinion, is to **eliminate caffeine.**

Numerous women have had successful results by this one change alone.

ALTERNATIVE CHOICES

- Nutrition - Vitamins – Minerals
- Progesterone Cream
- Herbs
- Exercise
- Castor Oil Packs
- Aromatherapy
- Affirmations

Nutrition – Vitamins – Minerals

Significantly reduce or **eliminate caffeine** from all sources, including coffee, colas, chocolate (we know how difficult this one is, so try taking extra magnesium to help). Reduce hydrogenated fats and oils as much as possible. Try the following supplements in addition to a good daily multiple vitamin and mineral:

- **Vitamin E – 800-1200 IU day**
- Vitamin B6 – 50 mg. day
- Additional Magnesium (in addition to the Calcium/Magnesium you may already be taking) – 250 to 300 mg. day
- Flax Seed Oil

Exercise

Exercise is great and works for almost all physical concerns, and it is especially helpful in this instance because it improves circulation and lymph drainage in the breast area. **Exercise daily if even for a few minutes.**

Progesterone Cream

Very good results using natural progesterone cream. Follow directions or try taking 1/4 to 1/2 teaspoon two times a day for the last two weeks of your cycle. See section on "Progesterone Creams."

Castor Oil Packs

See section on how to prepare "Castor Oil Packs." Feels wonderful!

Herbs

Red Clover, **Wild Yam,** Blessed Thistle, Echinacea, Goldenseal, Pau D'Arco

Try: Red Clover tea or Jason Winters Tea (which is primarily Red Clover)

Aromatherapy

Geranium, Jasmine, **Rose,** Rosewood

AFFIRMATIONS

I give and take nourishment in perfect balance.

I love being a woman.

My body is a beautiful temple for my spirit, and I am filled with the joy of living.

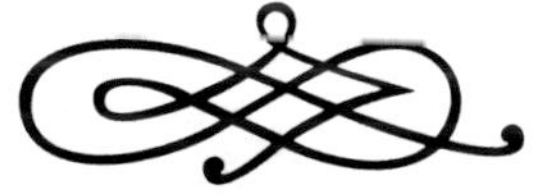

Fibroids

Fibroids are benign uterine growths which often go totally unnoticed until you have a routine pelvic exam. Fibroids are the number one reason for hysterectomy in this country. This is unusual because most fibroids are not cancerous.[3]

Fibroids most often attach to the inside of the uterus, and you may or may not have symptoms. If you do have symptoms they might include such things as menstrual cramps, pelvic pain, excessive bleeding, pelvic pressure, or frequent urination. Fibroids often fluctuate in size with your menstrual cycle or other stress factors. Hormone replacement and estrogen replacement can encourage growth or increase the size of fibroids.

Cause of fibroid growth is not really known, however, fibroids can run in families. Remedies include the surgical removal of only the fibroids (myomectomy) which is far less drastic than removal of the uterus (hysterectomy). On the other hand, it is often a good idea to just wait, if you can, because fibroids do shrink on their own, especially once a woman reaches menopausal years.

In addition, dietary changes are very successful in reducing fibroids. Other natural therapies such as relaxation, visualization, hypnosis, herbs, castor oil packs, and aromatherapy are also beneficial in reducing and eliminating fibroids.

ALTERNATIVES

- Nutrition – Vitamins – Minerals
- Herbs
- Visualization
- Castor Oil Packs
- Aromatherapy
- Affirmations

Nutrition – Vitamins – Minerals

Dietary changes are quite effective in ridding yourself of fibroids. Dr. Christiane Northrup who wrote *Women's Bodies, Women's Wisdom* suggests a diet similar to the following for women with fibroids.

- Eat a low fat (20%), high complex carbohydrate, mostly vegetarian diet
- Eliminate dairy, red meat, chicken and refined sugar
- Take a multiple vitamin/mineral supplement
- At least 600 mg. Magnesium and 1200 mg. Calcium
- B Complex Vitamins
- Vitamin C with Bioflavanoids 1000 to 3000 mg/day
- Floradex for iron – Do not take iron tablets

It is also a good idea to include the following into your lifestyle:

- Aerobic exercise twenty minutes three times per week
- Massage, Tai Chi, or Meditation are of great benefit

Castor Oil Packs

Apply castor oil pack to lower abdomen three times per week. See section on "Castor Oil Packs."

Herbs

Vitex or Chaste Tree – 20 to 30 drops in a tincture daily for two to three months

Red Clover – blood purifier and helps cleanse liver

Motherwort – restores thickness and moisture of vaginal walls

Echinacea – builds immune system

Valarian or Passion Flower – anti-inflammatory and for relaxation

Aromatherapy

Geranium – balances hormones and adrenals

Eucalyptus – disinfecting and helps with sore muscles

Chamomile – calming, stress reliever

Clary Sage – helps with cramps

Visualization

Visualizing your tumors shrinking and disappearing is very effective for fibroids. Deep relaxation such as breathing, meditating, or praying, along with visualization techniques when used together are powerful tools that encourage significant changes at the cellular level.

AFFIRMATIONS

I release old patterns and create only good in my future.

Today is a beautiful day which I choose to experience fully.

I accept and reclaim my own power.

Hair

Many women experience thinning or loss of hair at menopause. Baldness or loss of hair is known as *alopecia.* Hormones and mineral uptake are related to hair thinning and/or loss. Hair loss is also related to lifestyle, diet, and environmental conditions.

Conditions that contribute to this problem include:

- Vitamin or mineral deficiency
- Hormones, estrogen & progesterone
- Stress, tension
- Cancer treatments and drugs
- Sudden weight loss
- Iron deficiency
- Allergies
- Acute illness
- Heredity
- After pregnancy
- Poor circulation
- Thyroid disease

Hair loss can be a result of a drop in progesterone due to lack of ovulation. Some pregnant women have experienced hair loss a couple months after giving birth which may also be due to a sudden drop in progesterone that sometimes occurs at birth (known as post-partum depression).

Poor circulation adds to loss of hair. Itching and dry scalp are also common. Dry weather (especially in winter), drying hair products, allergic reactions to certain hair ingredients, or lack of moisture in the body can all contribute. To increase circulation to the hair, massage hot oil into your scalp. Yoga, especially postures that bring blood to the head, are effective.

An underactive thyroid, known as "hypothyroidism," influences loss of hair and is also recognized by fatigue and low temperature. At perimenopause or menopause, it is not uncommon for women to develop thyroid problems. Should this happen, be extra vigilant in paying attention to other potential perimenopausal or menopausal conditions along with improving your lifestyle (diet, stress, circulation, etc.) Be sure to check this out with your doctor. There are pharmaceutical drugs for the thyroid *and* there are natural solutions from herbs containing iodine or other ingredients which can be beneficial for thyroid as well.

Treat your head like the rest of your skin. Keep it clean, use healthy products, (perhaps purchasing shampoos and conditions that do not have sodium laureth sulfate), massage your head daily.

ALTERNATIVE CHOICES

- Nutrition – Vitamins – Minerals
- Progesterone Cream
- Aromatherapy
- Herbs
- Visualization
- Affirmations

Nutrition - Vitamins -Minerals

Biotin – either orally or topically

Vitamin C with Bioflavanoids – 1000 mg. or more

Vitamin E – 800 IU per day

Multiple Vitamins plus B Complex

Calcium/Magnesium – 1200 to 1500 mg. Day

Floradex – Liquid herbal iron tonic

HOT OIL TREATMENTS using olive or wheat germ oil. (Heat two tablespoons and massage into scalp. Wrap head with hot wet towel or sit in the sun with hair uncovered for about thirty minutes.)[4]

Herbs

Kelp – contains iodine and is helpful to thyroid

Horsetail – for thicker hair

HERBAL TEA HAIR RINSES help prevent your hair from falling out. Use marshmallow, rosemary, sage or nettles. Apple cider vinegar rinses can help your hair to grow.

Aromatherapy

Peppermint – stimulates scalp

Rosemary – for dandruff and alopecia

Progesterone Cream

Progesterone creams provide natural progesterone to the body which helps bring the estrogen and progesterone back into balance. See section on "Progesterone Creams" for more details.

AFFIRMATIONS

I have thick, beautiful hair.

My hair grows easily.

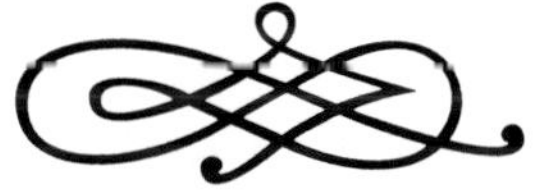

Headaches

Headaches and migraines often accompany perimenopause as well as menopause. Cyclical headaches are common just prior to menstruation or mid-cycle, and maybe you have already experienced this. A rise in estrogen just prior to menstruation is usually the cause. If you are premenstrual or have excess estrogen in your system from taking prescribed hormones, you too may experience headaches and/or migraines.

Estrogen is not the only hormone involved with headaches and migraines, however, it is believed that estrogen affects the serotonin activity in the brain. Serotonin is a natural pain reliever. If it is not available to do its job then you will experience headache pain. Menstrual disorders, often resulting from an imbalance or fluctuation between estrogen and progesterone, also cause headaches.

There are many other contributing factors to headaches including diet, environment, or stress related factors, and others which include:

- Caffeine and Chocolate
- Sugar
- Digestive Disturbances
- MSG
- Computer Screens
- Liver Toxicity
- High Blood Pressure
- Hypoglycemia
- Environmental
- Factors, such as Fluorescent Lights
- Muscular Constriction around Neck and Eyes
- Constipation
- Allergies
- Hangovers
- Stress and Tension
- Chemical Fumes
- Eyestrain
- Red Wine
- Poor Posture

Also see section on "Migraines."

ALTERNATIVE CHOICES

- Eliminate Estrogen Containing Drugs
- Progesterone Cream
- Nutrition – Vitamins – Minerals
- Herbs
- Aromatherapy
- Affirmations

Eliminate Estrogen Containing Drugs

If your headache or migraine began or are related to taking estrogen type drugs, it is probably a good idea to stop taking these. Drugs that contain estrogen include birth control pills, Premarin, and all forms of estrogen and progestin drugs.

Progesterone Cream

Progesterone creams provide natural progesterone to the body which helps bring the estrogen and progesterone back into balance. See section on "Progesterone Creams" for more details.

Nutrition – Vitamins – Minerals

Start to eliminate or, at least, cut back on the foods mentioned above such as caffeine, chocolate, red wine, and sugar. Make sure you are drinking enough water. You may also wish to add to your dietary plan:

- **Drink at least eight 8 oz. glasses of water daily**
- Vitamin C with Bioflavanoids – 1000 mg. or more
- Vitamin E – 800 IU per day
- Potassium – under 100 mg. per day
- Multiple Vitamins plus B Complex
- **Calcium/Magnesium** – 1200 to 1500 mg. day

Herbs

Valerian – relaxant

Passion Flower – acts as an anti-inflammatory

Feverfew – excellent for preventing migraines

Peppermint – for nausea

Burdock – cleanses liver

Cascara Sagrada – aid for constipation

TEAS: Chamomile, Hops

Aromatherapy

Peppermint, Lavender, Chamomile, Rosemary, Rosewood

AFFIRMATIONS

I release any and all negative energy and see only through the eyes of love.

My mind is refreshed and I am at peace.

I pay attention and honor all messages my body gives me.

Heart Disease

Heart disease is the number one killer of women over the age of fifty-five in America, and one in every three women will die from it. It is one of the main reasons, along with osteoporosis, women are encouraged to take estrogen replacement therapy at menopause. Although estrogen helps to increase the healthy cholesterol (HDL) and lower the bad cholesterol (LDL), no research has ever demonstrated a cause and effect relationship between a lack of estrogen and an increased risk of heart disease.[5] Additionally, no studies exist of older women who do not have heart disease and who are not taking estrogen.[6] Therefore, lack of estrogen does not cause heart disease!

When we talk about heart disease, we are talking about the kind of problem that exists when arteries narrow due to plaque build up. Plaque comes from cholesterol, but then all hormones, including estrogen, come from cholesterol too. Check your cholesterol level with your doctor periodically and avoid the "bad" fats. Bad fats are any hydrogenated and polyunsaturated oils including margarine and especially pre-packaged foods which often contain these fats. Go for olive oil, flax oil, all Omega 3 oils. Be sure to include natural butter instead of margarine because, although saturated, it has vitamins A, D, E, selenium, lecithin and has a healthy effect on the immune system[7]. Naturally, eat it in moderation.

Chances of developing heart disease are based on many other factors other than estrogen such as lifestyle, diet, exercise, and more.

Factors that can increase your chances of heart disease are:

> **High Fat Diet, High Sugar Consumption, Smoking, Stress, Diabetes, Obesity (more than 20% over target weight), High Blood Pressure, Sedentary Lifestyle, Genetics**

Heart disease is a serious concern and requires intervention with a doctor or physician. Alternatives suggested here are in addition to the direction of your health care provider. You may also wish to seek out a doctor who is practitioner of the "Dean Ornish Program," (which is rather expensive, yet effective).

ALTERNATIVE CHOICES

- Nutrition – Vitamins – Minerals
- Herbs
- Visualization
- Exercise
- Aromatherapy
- Affirmations

Nutrition – Vitamins – Minerals

- **If you smoke – quit now!**
- Eat more fiber, complex carbohydrates, whole grains, fresh fruits, and vegetables
- Lower fat and protein intake (especially red meat, pork, fried foods, fast foods)
- Reduce caffeine, sugar, table salt
- Reduce alcohol – although one glass of red wine per day claims to be helpful
- Avoid prepared, packaged and frozen dinner foods and learn to cook simple, nutritious meals (See section on "Nutrition" for more details)
- Take antioxidants – Vitamins A, C, E, and Selenium
- B complex vitamins essential – B6 helps lower cholesterol and prevents blood clots
- Vitamin C with Bioflavanoids – 1000 to 3000 mg./day
- Beta carotene and Omega 3's (flax oil, borage oil, fish oil – one tablespoon a day)

Exercise

Many good choices are available. Just move. Get your circulation going through your body. **Walking** is best and easiest. Start with a ten or twenty minute walk and increase your time and effort from there.

Herbs

Hawthorn – strengthens and regulates heart

Gingko & Cayenne – for circulation

Garlic – lowers cholesterol

Alfalfa – for minerals and lowers cholesterol

Motherwort – for heart palpitations

Valerian – calms nerves, reduces anxiety, tension

Peppermint tea – calms palpitations and is preventative

Parsley tea – heart toner

Aromatherapy

Lavender, Ylang Ylang, Rose, Lemon, Marjoram

Visualization

Relax, close your eyes and take several slow, deep breaths. Now imagine yourself at the sea shore. It is a beautiful, clear, pleasant day. Enjoy the sand beneath your bare feet and feel the warmth of the sun on your skin as you notice the waves lapping up on the shore, over and over, ever so gently. Allow yourself to become part of the rhythm of nature around you. Continue to breathe in and out with the gentle movement of the waves.

AFFIRMATIONS

I lovingly and peacefully allow joy to flow through my heart.

My heart beats with the rhythm of love.

My heart is strong and healty.

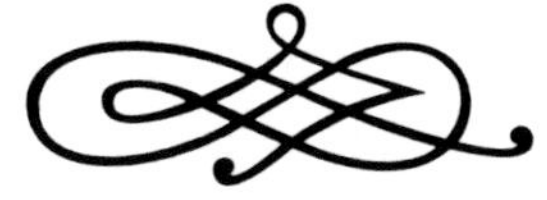

Heart Palpitations

As you enter and proceed through menopause, the hormonal change affects different parts of your body including the heart. This is a normal experience. Heart palpitations may be a result of fluid loss from hot flashes, cholesterol fluctuation, or stressful situations. Always be sure to seek professional help if your palpitations leave you extremely breathless, dizzy, in great pain, or should you have any other concerns. Remember, it's always advisable to have your cholesterol level checked regularly.

ALTERNATIVE CHOICES

- Nutrition – Vitamins – Minerals
- Herbs
- Relaxation
- Exercise
- Aromatherapy
- Affirmations

Nutrition – Vitamins – Minerals

- **Reduce Caffeine**
- Reduce Salt
- Drink eight 8 oz glasses of water daily
- Drink grape juice or eat some grapes
- **Take Supplemental Magnesium – 250 to 300 mg.**

Exercise

Moderate **exercise** keeps the heart muscle in shape. A couple deep breaths and a walk around the block calms you and increases circulation to all your muscles.

Herbs

Valerian – for nerves

Hawthorn – to strengthen heart

Motherwort – promotes blood circulation and eases palpitations

Aromatherapy

Lavender, Chamomile, Peppermint, Rose

Relaxation

Close your eyes, place one hand on your heart and the other on your solar plexus. Breath slowly for two to three minutes or until your heart is even and quiet. Breathe through your nose, taking slow deep breaths. As you exhale, tell yourself to melt and relax. You will actually feel your heart rate slow down.

AFFIRMATIONS

Be still and know that I am God.

My heart beats with the rhythm of love, peace and joy.

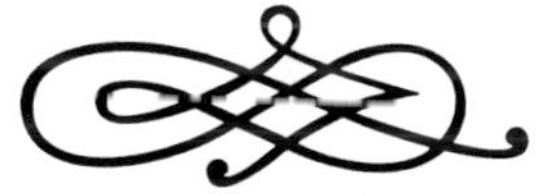

Heavy Bleeding

Heavy bleeding, also known as flooding, results when there is a sudden drop in progesterone which signals the uterus to contract and expel menses. Even if you have never experienced heavy bleeding, once you enter perimenopause or menopause, irregular periods are common and may include episodes of heavy bleeding, scanty bleeding, or clotted bleeding. Your cycle may also become more erratic and unpredictable, even skipping a month or two all together. *All of these symptoms are normal during perimenopause.*

For now, let's focus on heavy bleeding. Heavy bleeding is caused by erratic hormones and especially progesterone disturbance. It can also be an indication of fibroid tumors, ovarian cysts, infection, polyps or, in rare instances, cancer. Heavy loss of blood also means loss of iron which may contribute to weakness or dizziness, so it is important to keep iron levels high. However, be cautious of taking iron in tablet form or in vitamins. Iron is hard to digest, causes constipation and is not easily absorbed unless taken by way of foods or herbs. You may wish to try a liquid preparation called **Floradex** or Yellowdock herb.

If you are concerned about any of the conditions mentioned above or are experiencing persistent low back pain, regular pain upon intercourse, excessive weakness, dizziness or confusion, please consult a health professional. See the section on "Fibroids" also.

Heavy bleeding is aggravated by:

- Aspirin
- Fibroids
- Excessive Alcohol
- Lack of Exercise
- IUD's

Herbs are recommended throughout this guide and are wonderful alternatives to drugs and/or surgery. With heavy bleeding, there are certain herbs that need to be reduced or avoided. They are listed as herbs to curb or avoid on the following page, please take notice.

Hysterectomy is often recommended for heavy bleeding or for fibroids. It is the most over-prescribed, and often unnecessary, procedure for women. Realize that hysterectomy is a drastic step and not reversible! Please try several other remedies, if at all possible, before submitting to a hysterectomy.

ALTERNATIVE CHOICES

- Nutrition – Vitamins – Minerals
- Progesterone Cream
- Aromatherapy
- Herbs
- Castor Oil Packs
- Affirmations

Nutrition – Vitamins – Minerals

Be sure you are getting enough iron. Take iron in small doses, through food sources or herbs, throughout the day. Taken with orange juice or milk enhances absorption of iron. **Molasses** is a great source of iron and can be taken daily, used on cereals, or drink a teaspoon in milk.

FOODS TO AVOID: Caffeine, Coffee, Black Tea, Soy

Include In Diet:

- Calcium in smaller doses of about 250 mg.
- **Molasses**
- Vitamin C with Bioflavanoids
- B6 – 50 mg. or less
- EFA Oils (**Flax seed,** Borage, Black Currant or Primrose Oil)
- **Floradex** for Iron – do not take iron tablets

Progesterone Cream

Progesterone cream made from Wild Yam provides a safe source for progesterone. Follow directions on cream and please refer to section on "Progesterone Creams."

Castor Oil Packs

Apply castor oil packs to abdomen three times a week for two weeks prior to period.

Herbs

Dandelion – herbal iron and tones liver

Ginseng – helps regulate menses, nourishes glands

Sage – antispasmodic for pain and bleeding

Vitex – normalizes cycles, raises progesterone and estrogen, however, slow acting, must be taken over a period of months. (See section on "Herbs.")

Wild Yam – balances progesterone

Yellowdock – herbal iron source

CURB OR AVOID: Black Cohosh, Dong Quai, Motherwort, Red Clover, Alfalfa, Willowbark, Wintergreen

Aromatherapy

Cypress, **Geranium,** Lemon, Rose

AFFIRMATIONS

Joy flows through my body.

Love and peace fill my life in every precious moment.

Hot Flashes

Hot flashes are an acute symptom related to a drop in estrogen. When the ovaries no longer respond properly to the hormone signals from the pituitary, you experience a hot flash, night sweat, or a warm flush. Your ovaries may still be producing some estrogen, just not as much, and you may not be producing any progesterone. Consequently, estrogen and progesterone are out of balance, and your body is attempting to respond to the signals from the pituitary. The overactivity of the pituitary as it puts out more FSH, triggers other parts of the brain to respond in ways that result in hot flashes.

A hot flash is an attempt by the body to cool down. You may even get a warning just prior to a hot flash. If this happens, you can be prepared to help yourself cool down and stay comfortable by the clothes you wear, by carrying a fan or mini-electrical fan, and by always having cool water to drink (keep a bottle in the car with you when you drive). Signs of an imminent hot flash vary from woman to woman, but many say it's just a "knowing" from within. It might be accompanied by a tickling or other feeling, so tune in to your body's signals. Spicy foods, warm rooms, caffeine, and stress can also trigger hot flashes.

Remember, even if hot flashes go untreated, they are temporary. They are temporary in the moment, and they are temporary in that they only last over a short period of time. What that period of time is depends on the person (anywhere from a couple months to a couple years). Hot flashes continue until your body brings itself back into balance and adjusts to the hormonal changes. Certainly, the more you do to help your body adjust such as diet, relaxation, exercise (helps reduce FSH and LH), meditation, and herbs, the less discomfort you will have overall. In the meantime, acknowledge your flashes as part of you, then breathe, and "go with the flow" as best you can. Following are some good tips and ideas you may want to try.

ALTERNATIVE CHOICES

- Clothing
- Nutrition – Vitamin – Minerals
- Relaxation
- Herbs
- Aromatherapy
- Affirmations

Clothing

- **Wear Natural Fibers**
- Layer Your Look for Flexibility
- Buy Easy-Fitting Clothes

Cotton is a natural fiber that breathes and is a good choice. Polyesters are a problem because they don't breathe. It makes you cooler when you get cold and makes you warmer when you get hot. Natural fibers allow your body to adjust easier and more quickly to temperature changes. Silk is also a natural fiber which some women like. You may wish to start buying cotton underwear as well as sleepwear (especially helpful if you wake up with night sweats) and clothing. Also, stick with cotton sheets, blankets, and bedding.

Layer your clothes with removable jackets or sweaters for flexibility during weather changes (inside and out)! Wear clothes a little loose so they are comfortable, but not so loose it looks baggy. You'll know. Avoid tight, binding waists, legs or anything that restricts the body and doesn't let it breathe.

Nutrition – Vitamins – Minerals

- Eat a balanced diet and reduce Red Meat, Caffeine, Sugar and Alcohol
- Miso Soup (fermented soy product contains many healthy minerals)
- Increase Calcium/Magnesium to 2000/1000 mg/day[8]
- **Vitamin E 800 IU – increase as needed to 1200 IU**
- Flax Seed Oil – 1 Tablespoon a day or equivalent gel capsules (about 12 to 15)
- Bee Pollen – 500 mg./day

Herbs

Black Cohosh (very strong, best used in combination herb products or in homeopathic strength)

Dong Quai, Damiana, Ginseng, Sage, Vitex

Remifemin® (herbal remedy from Germany; base is black cohosh; recommended for six months of use only)

Aromatherapy

Clary Sage, **Geranium**, Chamomile, Lavender, Grapefruit, Ylang Ylang

Relaxation

Take a moment to just close your eyes and stop what you're doing. Now, take a couple of slow, deep breaths and focus in your heart area. As you do this, visualize the heat that's running through you turning into the warmth of love. Send the love throughout your body and imagine the peace and harmony it brings to all levels of your being, physical, mental, emotional, and spiritual.

AFFIRMATIONS

Loving energy flows throughout my body.

I am empowered.

I am transformed by my energy.

Migraines

Migraines are headaches, but more intense. Women are more likely candidates to suffer from migraines than are men. The intensity of a migraine can disable a person to the point of causing nausea, blurred vision, diarrhea, even tingling or numb sensations in the hands or feet.

Migraines can be triggered by several things including hypoglycemia (low blood sugar), hormone fluctuations and imbalance (primarily excess estrogen in comparison to progesterone), stress, constipation, digestive disorders, poor circulation, eyestrain, candida, head and neck injuries.

Food sensitivities are also recognized as a source of migraines. Approximately twenty-five percent of all migraines are food related.

Some foods that can trigger migraines include:

- Aspartame artificial sweeteners
- Cured meats, i.e. ham, bacon, etc.
- Citrus Fruits
- MSG
- Nightshade family, i.e. tomatoes, potatoes, eggplant, peppers
- Aged cheeses
- Yogurt
- Red Wine
- Chocolate
- Candida

If you are a person who has experienced migraines throughout your life, the good news is that migraines often disappear when you reach menopause. Not always true, however. Massage is helpful for circulation and relaxation.

I have heard more than one account where pulling on your hair, or having someone do this for you, can release pain and energy from the head and relieve a migraine. Actually, this feels very good. Take a handful of hair and pull gently, yet firmly, then release and take another handful of hair. Repeat this all over the head for several minutes or more.

ALTERNATIVE CHOICES

- Nutrition – Vitamins – Minerals
- Progesterone Cream
- Herbs
- Aromatherapy
- Relaxation
- Affirmations

Nutrition – Vitamins – Minerals

Determine and reduce or avoid the aggravating food items as listed above. Follow a good, basic nutritional program as described in the section on "Nutrition." Additionally, you may wish to try:

- **Supplemental Magnesium – 300 mg./day**
- **Vitamin B6**
- Odorless Garlic
- Niacin – 50 to 100 mg. to dilate blood vessels to head. You should experience a niacin flush (this does not occur with niacinamide) which is like a rush of blood to the skin surface.

Progesterone Cream

If excess estrogen or estrogen dominance is related to your migraines, use natural progesterone cream daily or as per directions. See section on "Progesterone Creams."

Herbs

Feverfew – A relaxant which is a good preventative taken daily

Gingko Biloba – Improves circulation to head

Valerian – For pain and as a sedative

Passion Flower – Muscle relaxing

Peppermint – For nausea and headache

Dong Quai – Used daily can be a preventative

Wild Yam – Helps balance hormones

TEAS: Hops, Red Clover, Chamomile

Aromatherapy

Any of the scents may be used to permeate the air. Rub a drop at temples, between the eyes and on back of neck. Try massaging it on your toes too.

- **Lavender or Chamomile** – relaxing and calming
- Peppermint – uplifting and settles nausea
- Geranium – a sweet fragrance for balancing hormones

Relaxation

Take a cool compress (or washcloth with one drop of aromatherapy fragrance) and place it over your eyes. Rest and lay down for as long as needed. Do slow, deep breathing making your belly balloon out on the in breath and relaxing out as you exhale. Imagine releasing any tension or pain as you breathe out.

AFFIRMATIONS

I relax, let go and flow with life.

I accept and adapt easily to change.

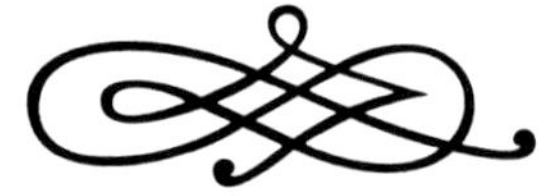

Osteoporosis

Osteoporosis affects eight million Americans and eighty percent of those are older women.[9] Osteoporosis is the progressive loss of bone mass and bone strength often associated with menopause. However, osteoporosis does not just happen at menopause nor is menopause the only factor.

Bone loss does not automatically start at perimenopause or menopause. Around the age of thirty to thirty-five and older, we begin to lose bone at a rate of .5 to 1.5% per year. You may have learned that once you lose bone, there is no way to get it back. This is not true. There are many ways to prevent bone loss as well as increase bone density no matter what your age. It has been proven that seniors between the ages of seventy and eighty were still able to rebuild bone with exercise and nutrition. Natural progesterone creams are also excellent for helping regenerate bone.

Estrogen replacement (ERT) is promoted as a preventative therapy for osteoporosis, however, osteoporosis is not an estrogen deficiency condition, and this is being challenged in recent studies. There are many other factors which affect bone density and include stress, smoking, drug intake, nutrition, lack of exercise, calcium, and other mineral deficiencies. It has been shown that estrogen slows bone loss for a few years, but its effect tapers off soon after menopause, and estrogen does not rebuild new bone. In addition, estrogen replacement therapy has negative side effects. Natural alternatives do not. Before accepting an estrogen replacement drug, please consider other alternatives available that *prevent* additional bone loss and *rebuild* bone.

Preventing bone loss earlier, rather than later, is the ideal situation. Substances that contribute towards bone loss and which you may want to use in moderation or eliminate completely are:

> **Caffeine, Sodas, Excessive Protein Especially Red Meat, Tobacco, Cortisone Drugs Including Prednizone, Steroids, Diuretics, Antacids Containing Aluminum, Excessive Alcohol Consumption, and Lack of Weight Bearing Exercise.**

Be sure to ask for a Bone Mineral Density (BMD) test from your doctor to determine your bone density prior to or immediately upon reaching menopause to have a baseline. You may have to request this because it is not always automatically offered. Also, check if your insurance covers this test which it may not. Even if it's not covered under your insurance, pay for it yourself because it is a very important test to have done. There are several ways to test the bones, ask which uses less x-rays. The DPA or DEXA tests are the ones recommended by Dr. John R. Lee.

Certainly, some women are more prone to develop osteoporosis than others. Please take a look at and fill out the following chart on "Your Risk of Osteoporosis" to determine your risk level. It is a guideline only and not to be used in place of a BMD or other medical advice.

Alternatives exist that will stop and/or inhibit bone loss, and some of these same remedies actually help rebuild bone. These alternatives may require a little more initiative and activity on your part but they're safe and definitely well worth the effort.

ALTERNATIVE CHOICES

- Nutrition – Vitamins – Minerals
- Progesterone Cream
- Herbs
- Weight Bearing Exercise
- Affirmations

Nutrition - Vitamins - Minerals

Good digestion and assimilation is required along with a healthy diet to keep bones strong so you can absorb minerals. After all if you are not digesting and assimilating your foods and supplements, they won't be of much use. Digestive aids are available. Look for papaya, peppermint and acidophilus supplements. Other combination products with digestive enzymes are also helpful. **Please, no antacids, they actually inhibit digestion and are not good for you.**

Eat a diet rich in leafy green vegetables, fruits, whole grains, beans, legumes, yogurt and soy products, especially miso. **Eliminate soft drinks** and reduce your intake of caffeine, sugar, processed foods, colas, fluoridated water, and red meat. Re-evaluate your need for drugs, especially cortisone drugs. Use meditation, breathing, and other relaxation techniques to reduce stress in your life.

Digestion is important to adequately process and absorb calcium. To aid digestion and also to add potassium and minerals to the body, the following digestive aid is one you can prepare at home. Take this fifteen minutes before a meal and up to three times a day.

In a 6 oz. glass of water add:

1 tsp. Apple Cider Vinegar (organic preferably)

1 tsp. Honey

You May Also Wish To Add To Your Nutritional Program:

- **1000 - 1500 mg. of Calcium/Magnesium supplement** (Read thoroughly the section on "Calcium/Magnesium" for types of supplements and how to take).
- B-Complex (extra B6 and B12)
- Vitamin C with Bioflavanoids – aids assimilation of Calcium
- Vitamin D (do not overdue; getting out in the sun for 10 min. a day is sufficient)
- Vitamin E
- Potassium, Silicon, Sulfur

Progesterone Cream

Natural progesterone creams encourage bone regeneration. Use cream as per directions and see section on "Progesterone Creams."

Herbs

Many herbs are very high in calcium and magnesium, and often herbs are easier to digest and assimilate that vitamins. Look for capsules rather than compressed or coated tablets. You may wish to try these herbs:

Alfalfa	Horsetail	Kelp	Oatstraw
Red Clover	Slippery Elm	Valerian	

Weight Bearing Exercise

Weight bearing exercise encourages bone rebuilding and keeps them strong too. The stress of weight on the bones encourages bone regeneration, and with a little effort you can accomplish more than you realize no matter what your age.

- **Walking** is the best and easiest weight bearing exercise to do.
- Resistance training, weight training and lifting are good.
- Other exercises that fulfill weight bearing are tennis, volleyball, basketball, jogging.
- Stretching is excellent, helps flexibility and increases circulation to bones and muscles.
- Get a mini-trampoline you can store under a bed and use it daily. It's easy on the joints, great for circulation in addition to being an excellent weight-bearing exercise.

Other exercises that are helpful and very popular today include yoga and tai chi. Although these are not considered weight-bearing, they assist in flexibility, circulation, and relaxation. You can learn these at a class or there are many videos you can purchase and learn at home. See section on "Exercise."

AFFIRMATIONS

My life supports me.

I stand strong, I feel strong, I am strong.

I am building more strength, courage, and power into my life every day.

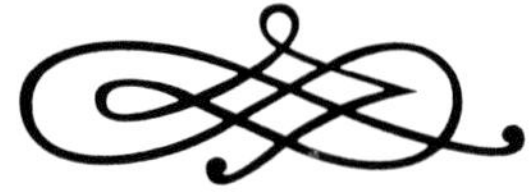

Your Risk of Osteoporosis

Following are factors that affect your chances of developing osteoporosis. Check the ones that apply to you. The more check marks you have, the more at risk you are of developing osteoporosis. No matter what your age, take the time you need to make healthy changes.

If you are concerned or just want to be careful, now is the best time to incorporate *lifestyle* changes to help prevent osteoporosis. Changes can be made in diet, exercise, calcium/magnesium supplements, and reducing any aggravating factors such as smoking, alcohol, etc. If you already have osteoporosis, be sure to include the suggestions provided in this guide. Also take a Calcium/Magnesium supplement that has microcrystalline hydroxyapatite (see section of "Calcium - Magnesium."

RISK FACTOR	SCORE
Smoking	________
Lack of weight bearing exercise	________
Family history of osteoporosis	________
Small, fine-boned frame	________
Caucasian or Asian racial background	________
Excessive consumption of protein, salt, alcohol, caffeine, soft drinks	________
First menstrual period after age 17	________
Long-term use of cortisone drugs	________
Calcium deficiency during adolescence and/or while nursing a child	________
Excessive exercise, especially if you develop amenorrhea (lack of menstruation)	________
Overactive thyroid	________
Amenorrhea (lack of menstruation for):	
6 to 12 months	________
12 to 14 months	________
2 to 5 years	________
5 to 10 years	________

The most accurate way to determine your risk is to have a bone mineral density test (BMD) done at the time of perimenopause or better yet, get a baseline reading before you enter perimenopause. A BMD can determine the density and the strength of your bones. The more dense your bones, the more resistant to fracture.

A BMD should be a routine screening test for all menopausal women. If your doctor does not suggest one, be sure to ask for it.

PMS

Premenstrual Syndrome, known to most people as PMS, may not be the first thing you think about when you think of menopause. However, PMS is a classic indication of hormonal imbalance and, usually, too much estrogen. Symptoms of PMS are suspiciously similar to some perimenopause and menopause symptoms.

PMS is not a specific malady, but rather it is a collection of symptoms that occur anywhere from a few days to two weeks prior to your period. You might experience one or more of the following:

- Bloating
- Anger
- Cravings
- Headaches
- Sore Breasts
- Constipation
- Weight gain
- Fatigue
- Irritability
- Confusion
- Depression
- Emotional Upheaval

Although, there are no laboratory tests to confirm if you have PMS, you know if you have it. PMS can get worse or more intense as you approach perimenopause. While progesterone should be the dominant hormone prior to your period, it seems that women with PMS tend to have lower progesterone levels than normal for that time of their cycle.

Other conditions can contribute to or aggravate PMS symptoms. For example, low thyroid causes fatigue and headaches, and yet, too much estrogen impairs thyroid function as well. The best way to determine if you have a low thyroid is to get a blood test to determine your thyroid levels.

Another factor is adrenal exhaustion which contributes to fatigue, unstable blood sugar, moodiness, foggy thinking, and more. Adrenals are important because they assist in producing hormones when the ovaries slow down. As mentioned throughout this book, it is very important to keep your adrenals healthy. They are the "fight or flight" gland and, unfortunately, stressful lifestyles often burn them out much too soon.

Nutrition and elimination are very important. Once the body is through using estrogen, it is eliminated through the intestines. If you do not get enough fiber in your diet, estrogen gets recirculated and reabsorbed instead of eliminated. Also, **estrogen increases fat and helps retain water.** This is why many beef and poultry are fed estrogens to fatten them up for market. Then, of course, we eat these. If you eat meat and poultry, look for estrogen-free whenever possible, and eat more vegetables and grains.

ALTERNATIVE CHOICES

- Nutrition – Vitamins – Minerals
- Progesterone Cream
- Reflexology
- Herbs
- Aromatherapy
- Affirmations

Nutrition - Vitamins – Minerals

- Eat a low fat (20%), fiber-rich diet
- Include grapes, cucumbers, asparagus, corn, watermelon to help relieve water retention
- Reduce fat, sugar, salt, caffeine, alcohol
- Calcium/Magnesium – double the amount at PMS time
- B Complex Vitamins, especially B6 – 50 mg.
- Supplemental Magnesium – 250 to 300 mg.
- Vitamin E – 400 to 800 IU

Progesterone Cream

Progesterone creams can be very helpful. Follow directions on the package insert. Usually 1/4 to 1/2 tsp. once or twice a day used during the second half of cycle; increase or decrease as needed. See section on "Progesterone Creams."

Herbs

Dandelion – for water retention

Nettles – for water retention and to nourish kidneys and adrenals

Dong Quai – relieves bloating

Cascara Sagrada – relieves constipation

St. John's Wort – for depression

Valerian – calms nerves, sedative and helps sleep

Wild Yam – balances hormones

TEAS: Hops, Red Clover, Chamomile, Dong Quai

Aromatherapy

Lavender, Chamomile – calms and balances

Grapefruit – for edema, weight gain, lifts moods

Geranium – helps balance hormones

Reflexology

According to a study done in 1993, thirty-five women with PMS showed reduction of symptoms up to forty percent by using reflexology.[10] Use aromatherapy oils on feet, especially at ankles along with this wonderful treatment. See section on "Reflexology."

AFFIRMATIONS

My hormones are in perfect working order.

I am happy in my body.

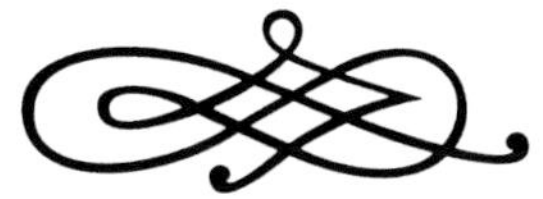

Skin

Wrinkles, aging, and mid-life acne (caused by hormonal upheaval) are the major concerns for women about their skin. Our modern lifestyle contributes to the problem, and therefore, lifestyle adjustments or improvements can also improve the look of your skin.

First of all, those things that cause wrinkles, aging, or lines include:

- Alcohol
- Poor Skin Care
- Smoking
- Lack of Internal and External Moisture
- Air Pollutants
- Prescription Medications
- Stress
- Poor Diet
- Overexposure to Sun

You cannot change the march of time, however, you can take care of your skin and improve your habits in order to manage the stresses and strains of our modern lifestyle. Proper diet, exercise and skin hydration will alleviate many of your concerns. It is important to take care of your skin from the *inside* (from what you eat and drink) as well as from the *outside* (how you clean and nourish your skin).

ALCOHOL is also very drying to the skin, disrupts the hormonal balance in your body, has no nutrition, inhibits your body from absorbing minerals and vitamins.

SMOKING is very harsh on your skin, partly because it is very drying as well as toxic. Smokers age and develop lines and wrinkles much earlier and quicker than non-smokers. Of course, it aggravates so many other conditions, including depleting calcium from your system. There are many ways to quit smoking, but first, you must decide for yourself and then commit to yourself, "it's time to stop." If you're a smoker, promise yourself you will quit, set a "deadline" date in which to do so, and then do it! I've met many people who've been successful in quitting by using patches, gum or hypnotherapy, and some who are able to quit "cold" turkey. If you can quit on your own, that's great. If you need assistance, then get it.

FORMICATION: A skin problem, you may have experienced and yet not known the name, is formication. Formication (from the Latin word for ant "formica") is a prickly, itchy sensation on the arms or legs which is caused by estrogen reduction. When estrogen drops, an over-worked, and over-heated liver aggravates this problem. For instant relief, a midwife suggests eating raw beets, grated or juiced, three times in one day.[11]

ALTERNATIVE CHOICES

- Nutrition – Vitamins – Minerals
- Herbs
- Aromatherapy
- Exercise
- Visualization
- Affirmations

Nutrition – Vitamins – Minerals

- **Eat a Balanced Diet including fresh fruits and vegetables**
- **Drink at least eight 8 oz. glasses of water daily to hydrate skin**
- Vitamin A and Carotenes
- B Complex Vitamins
- Vitamin C with Bioflavanoids
- Vitamin E internally AND Vitamin E Oil on skin for scars
- Omega 3 Oils – from Flaxseed oil, Borage oil, Primrose oil
- Zinc Oxide – a cream to protect, soothe, and heal skin
- **Always Use a Sunscreen – under makeup or in the sun**

Herbs

Dandelion – nourishes liver

Vitex or Chaste Tree – helps balance hormones

Chamomile – soothes skin

Aromatherapy

Sandalwood – Diminishes wrinkles and stimulates cell regeneration

Tea Tree – kills fungal and viral infections, and helps acne

Lavender – soothes and heals burns, irritations, acne

Exercise

Exercise improves circulation, reduces stress, helps remove toxins from the tissues and is helpful for all concerns of the skin. Improved circulation brings nutrients and oxygen to the skin.

Visualization

Visualization is extremely effective for any skin condition, including acne, rashes, and more. Sit back, relax your breathing, and imagine a healing color. If you have a "hot" skin condition, use a cool color such as blue or green to soothe. If you have a "cool" skin condition, use a warmer color such as yellow or orange to bring warmth to the area. It's a good idea to do this several times a day for a couple minutes each time until the condition improves or disappears.

AFFIRMATIONS

My skin is smooth and clear.

I love my body with exercise and good nutrition.

Sleep Disorders & Fatigue

Sleep disturbances include insomnia, night sweats, chills, hot flashes, having difficulty falling to sleep or waking up just after falling asleep, and remaining awake for some time. These disturbances cause you to get less rest and when you don't get enough rest, you find yourself tired and already on the road to fatigue the following day. Take heart, if you normally do not have trouble sleeping, then generally, these things are short-lived.

Night sweats are when you awaken in the middle of the night feeling hot and clammy. Some women claim they have "soaked" the sheets from sweating so profusely. Night sweats are really just hot flashes that occur while you are sleeping. They can be so intense as to awaken you, and then you may experience chills as your body attempts to cool down after the hot flash or night sweat.

Women may also notice sore muscles or leg cramps during the night. This is a classic symptom of a lack of proper calcium. Get enough calcium and magnesium by taking a balanced supplement, especially before bed, and eating more healthy throughout the day. This problem will disappear very quickly.

Stress, lack of exercise, caffeine, and alcohol contribute to restless sleep. **Exercise is one of the best remedies!** Take a walk, do some leg lifts, jump on a mini-trampoline, or just get enough exercise throughout the day. This alone can provide a better, more sound night's sleep.

Be cautious of pharmaceutical sleeping aids because they do not allow a natural sleep cycle, and you simply won't awaken feeling rested. For all sleep disorders, there are a number of natural remedies you can try before resorting to a drug. Melatonin is a fairly new supplement that people claim has provided good results and seems to work especially well for jet lag. However, some people have experienced negative side-effects with Melatonin, especially nightmares, so be aware should you decide to try this product. Use it only for a few days at a time,en and stop taking it if you experience any problems whatsoever.

A sound, restful sleep is essential to a healthy mind, body, and spirit, as well as energy! Sleep is when your body restores, repairs, heals, and integrates information and experiences. Keep a dream log during this transitional time, and you may find yourself more inspired than you've ever been.

ALTERNATIVE CHOICES

- Good Sleep Habits
- Sleeping Conditions
- Relaxation Techniques
- Herbs
- Aromatherapy
- Affirmations

Good Sleep Habits

- Herb teas, such as chamomile, help you relax before bed
- Reduce or eliminate caffeine especially before bed
- Do not eat heavy foods or meals at least three hours before bed
- Do not drink alcohol for sleep purposes
- Reduce sodium intake throughout the day
- Take B Complex Vitamins and especially Vitamin B6
- **Take an aromatherapy bath (use Lavender or Chamomile)**
- Listen to soothing music
- Write in a journal
- Go to bed around the same time each night
- Before bed do not stimulate your body or your brain with exercise, reading the newspaper, catching up on work, or watching the news

Sleeping Conditions

CLOTHING: Wear loose fitting, light-weight sleepwear. Cotton blends allow your body to breathe, whereas synthetic fibers increase and retain body heat.

BEDDING: Get rid of silk and flannel sheets and stick with cotton blends. Cotton thermal blankets are versatile because they keep you warm you when it's cold, and yet, they allow your body to breathe when you're warm.

ROOM CONDITIONS: Keep a window open for circulation and remember to set your thermostat to 68 degrees or lower.

Herbs

Valerian, Black Cohosh, Nettles, St. John's Wort, Sage, Motherwort

TEA: Ginseng – overall tonic for energy and balancing; do not take before bed.

Aromatherapy

Lavender, Chamomile, Clary Sage, Geranium

Relaxation Techniques

As you lay in a comfortable position in bed, place one of your hands over your lower abdomen area. Now breathe slowly and deeply while expanding your belly outwards on the "in" breath and relaxing your belly back on the "out" breath. With your hand you can feel the gentle rise and fall of your breath. With your eyes closed, focus on your muscles and notice how they begin to relax. Keep doing this until your whole body lets go of any tension or stress.

AFFIRMATIONS

My body rests easily throughout the night.

Peace and love circulate and sooth my body as I sleep.

I awaken each day feeling vibrant and energized.

Stress, Moodiness, Anxiety

Stress is part of life. Change is part of life. Perimenopause and menopause create unique hormonal changes which are stressful. Stress is also experienced in normal day-to-day living, and it cannot be avoided. Something as simple as boredom can cause stress. However, it is more likely to be caused by our jobs, by our personal and/or professional relationships, or from physical conditions. How much stress and how well we handle it varies from person to person. Some are more sensitive than others, and therefore, need to take more precautions to prevent stress. We all need to nourish and strengthen our physical, mental, and emotional bodies as well as our immune system in order to handle stress and stay healthy.

Lack of focus or concentration experienced under stress leads to mental or emotional problems, and if not resolved, may subsequently lead to burnout. Stress is a factor in mood swings, fatigue, memory loss, confusion, anxiety, panic, foggy thinking, depression, and other minor psychological disturbances. These can contribute to physical illness as well. When overloaded by stress, our immune system is weakened, which in turn manifests through illness, allergies, diseases, mental and emotional problems, even break downs.

Preventing stress is the ideal remedy, but not always practical. A little stress is actually good because it keeps us "on our toes" so to speak. The line between a "little" stress and "too much" stress is different for everyone. In order to reduce stress to an acceptable level for yourself, it is good to know what things contribute to your stress. You may already know, but here are some things to consider:

- Smoking
- Alcohol
- Obsessing about exercise
- Inner tension
- Chemotherapy
- Withdrawal from drugs, including estrogen
- Caffeine
- Lack of exercise
- Sugar
- Worry
- Personal crisis
- Family crisis

Exercise is a great stress buster! Again not enough emphasis can be placed on moving your body to help release tension and anxiety from your muscles, which in turn, improves circulation and lymph drainage. This allows your mind to relax at the same time.

Yoga and tai chi are excellent for the body and the mind. Relaxation, deep breathing, and inner reflection help us take control of stress and react to it in healthier ways. Just getting some sun every day also helps. We all handle stress in different ways, so pick one remedy that appeals to you and stick with it for awhile.

ALTERNATIVE CHOICES

- Nutrition – Vitamins – Minerals
- Aromatherapy
- Visualization
- Herbs
- Relaxation
- Affirmations

Nutrition – Vitamins – Minerals

Refer to the section on "Nutrition" for guidelines on healthy eating. Make sure you are getting adequate amounts of calcium/magnesium. You may also incorporate:

- Additional Magnesium – 300 mg. day
- **Vitamin C with Bioflavanoids – 2,000 to 3,000 mg.**
- B Complex Vitamins – at least 50 mg. of each

Herbs

St. John's Wort, Valerian, Passion Flower, Chamomile,

Aromatherapy

Lavender, **Geranium,** Chamomile, Grapefruit, Pine

Relaxation Techniques

Relaxation can be achieved in many ways, for example a few you can try are:

Meditation, yoga, hypnosis, biofeedback, massage, prayer, deep breathing, aromatherapy baths, listening to soft music, and, of course, exercise!

Listen to your intuition. To help you stay focused and concentrate in any situation, remain calm, centered and balanced as best you can, especially in times of stress.

Visualization

While in a relaxed state, visualize yourself sitting on a beautiful tropical beach. Feel the sand beneath your feet as you gaze out on the blue/green ocean. The waves make little lapping sounds as they flutter in. Notice the balmy air and the pleasantly warm sun on your skin. Now, slowly breathe in, and let this vision circulate through your veins bringing a peaceful feeling of calm and love to every cell of your body.

AFFIRMATIONS

The joy of life circulates through my veins.

Peace, love, and joy reside in my body.

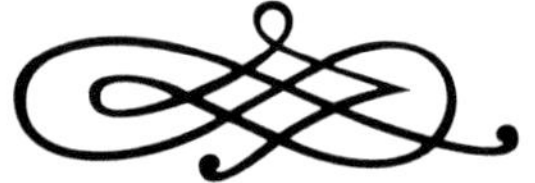

Vaginal Dryness, Atrophy, Infections

Vaginal dryness, atrophy, and infections are conditions many women experience at menopause. It is a common complaint, yet according to studies, it seems to occur in less than half the women going through menopause.[12] Furthermore, vaginal dryness is not unique to menopause, however, change in hormones and reduction of estrogen does affect the vaginal tissues. The vaginal wall becomes thinner, less resilient, and there is less mucus production, consequently you experience vaginal dryness, vaginal atrophy, and infections. These can all be resolved naturally.

Signs you may notice as your vaginal tissues start to thin include dryness, itching, pain on intercourse, vaginal or bladder infections, and less tone in the vaginal muscles. Vaginal atrophy or muscle weakness can be due to inactivity as well as to the hormonal changes. **Kegel exercises** are excellent for toning both the vaginal and bladder muscles.

Sometimes after a woman goes through the menopausal and perimenopausal years, vaginal dryness may or may not continue to be a problem. However, in the meantime, there are a number of remedies you can try for dryness, atrophy, or infections.

ALTERNATIVE CHOICES

- Nutrition – Vitamins – Minerals
- Douche
- Aromatherapy
- Affirmations
- Creams
- Herbs
- Kegel Exercises

Nutrition – Vitamins – Herbs

Eating a balanced diet with less caffeine, sugar, alcohol and carbohydrates is helpful for all conditions. Also try supplementing with the following:

- Vitamin B6 – 50 mg once or twice daily

- Magnesium – 300 mg. day
- Vitamin C with Bioflavanoids – 1000 to 5000 mg.
- Vitamin E – 400-800 IU – Can be used externally too for itching OR AS A LUBRICANT!
- **Acidophilus** – to regenerate the good intestinal flora. Take on empty stomach fifteen to thirty minutes prior to meals
- Flax Seed Oil – 1 Tablespoon a day

Creams

In addition to vaginal lubricants purchased over the counter, there are prescription vaginal creams and gels containing hormones. These creams are used intravaginally and are absorbed through the mucus membranes. If you decide to use a prescription remedy, ask your doctor for a **cream containing estriol.** Estriol is the least potent of the estrogens and is quite effective and safe.

Progesterone cream has also been found to be very helpful. Progesterone cream is used topically on the skin, not intravaginally (See section on "Progesterone Creams.") Used over a period of at least three or more months, women experience less vaginal dryness and fewer vaginal and urinary infections.[13] Some creams are made to be used vaginally as well.

Douche

Douching is quite helpful for infections. If you are taking antibiotics, remember to add acidophilus to restore the beneficial bacteria (this can be taken internally and used as a douche as well). Douche with one tablespoon of apple cider vinegar and water, or use one tablespoon of acidophilus to a quart of water. Try alternating these two douches for a week. Douching should not be done daily except for a short period of time. Be sure to check with your doctor if you are concerned or experiencing pain.

Herbs

Motherwort – to restore thickness and moisture

Echinacea/Goldenseal – for infections

Pau D'Arco – for candida

Oatstraw – high magnesium, helps infections;
Garlic - immune stimulant

Teas: Raspberry, Pau D'Arco, Oatstraw

Aromatherapy

Tea Tree – can also be used as a douche or in a bath for infections

Lavender, Bergamot, Eucalyptus

Kegel Exercises

For instruction on how to do Kegel exercises, please refer to the steps outlined under the section on "Bladder."

AFFIRMATIONS

I rejoice in being a woman.

My body is a temple of light and love.

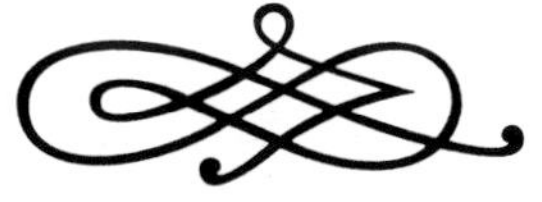

Weight Gain

Weight gain is one of the greatest concerns of women period! It's an even bigger concern with women in menopause or perimenopause.

MYTH: Menopause is the reason you gain weight.

FACT: Imbalanced hormones is the reason you gain weight.

Menopause itself does not cause significant weight gain. In 1992, the *International Journal of Obesity* stated there was no serious difference found between pre- and post-menopausal women with regard to total body weight, body mass index, waist-hip ratio, or total abdominal fat tissue. Hurray!

So what's the deal? Can you balance hormones prior to, during and after menopause. Yes, you can. It takes a little more involvement on your part. Why? Because weight concerns at perimenopause, menopause, and postmenopause require that you evaluate your lifestyle, your diet, your habits, your perspective on life, and yourself in general. Perimenopause, menopause, and postmenopause are times of transformation and a glorious re-awakening to one's true self and inner wisdom.

There are hundreds, if not thousands, of books and articles on weight and diets. There is far more extensive information than is even possible to mention here. However, believe and know that your weight is manageable. Should you gain a significant amount of weight during one period of time, review what happened just prior to that event, and your physical and emotional reaction to it. There may be other things to consider.

Many women put on weight when they start taking estrogen replacement therapy or birth control pills, however, there are always other factors to consider. Using synthetic or manufactured drugs is very harsh on your body and does affect weight. The goal is to listen to your body, treat it with kindness, and nourish it in healthy, natural ways. Feel and be aware of what is going on inside. Pay attention to your emotions, your gut, and any physical signs of change going on inside your body.

Really, *pay attention!* Your body will tell you everything you need to know.

Some believe it is a good idea to have extra fat at menopause because after the ovaries slow down, some estrogen is manufactured in your fat. Fat can increase the estrogen levels, but this may or may not be what you want depending on the individual situation. Information seems to support the fact that women in menopause, for the most part, have enough estrogen but not enough progesterone. Again it is the balance between estrogen and progesterone that causes many problems including weight gain.

ALTERNATIVE CHOICES

- Personal Weight Inventory
- Aromatherapy
- Herbs
- Visualization
- Affirmations

Personal Weight Inventory

- **Pay attention** to what point in your cycle you gain weight or when you have the most difficulty balancing your weight. Start working with a health professional to balance your hormone levels, and your weight problem will also start to come into balance.
- **If you are taking drugs of any kind, find out if any of them are affecting your weight** and what, if any, alternatives you have. Possibly consider reducing or eliminating the drugs, but check with your doctor first. Also read and do your own research because many doctors are not aware of, or informed about, natural alternatives and especially herbs, or homeopathics.
- **Learn to take care of your body.** Get a massage, learn yoga or tai chi, meditate, learn breathing relaxation techniques, experiment with herbs, herbal remedies, teas and even aromas.
- **Determine if you are eating out of physical hunger, stress, or emotional hunger.** Then be willing to make changes or try new approaches to release the negative behavior and develop healthier habits.

- **Nurture yourself in positive ways.** Take bubble baths, read a good book or work on your favorite hobby. Make a list of all the non-food activities you like to do. Post it on your refrigerator, and make a pact with yourself to do one thing each day! It can be as simple as petting your dog, smelling the flowers, gardening or savoring a nice hot cup of herbal tea while you listen to music.
- **Follow a healthy, nutritional eating program.** Any of the nutritional guidelines in this book are helpful. Read books on nutrition and design your own eating plan. No one specific diet works for everyone, so determine what works best for you and what you like, or consult a nutritionist who can advise you.
- Find a good **support group**, network or, better yet, start your own. I designed a very effective weight loss program using specific motivational techniques in a group environment. The group support was one of the major factors in helping people lose weight.
- **Journal.** Keep a daily journal of your eating habits and how you feel when you eat. Journal about anything else that is on your mind. **Fact:** People who journal are much healthier and happier than people who don't. Get a notebook and start putting your thoughts and ideas on paper today.
- **Exercise** every day. Just five minutes of walking brings benefits; do more when possible. Find something that appeals to you. Rebounding on a mini-trampoline is extremely helpful for circulation, lymph drainage, relaxation, and can be done right in your own home. Walk for ten, fifteen, or twenty minutes and notice how great you feel! Also see section on "Exercise" for more tips.
- Make sure your **digestive system and elimination systems are working well.** Take a good digestive enzyme product or try the Cider Vinegar recipe to improve digestion and assimilation. Make sure you have regular, daily bowel movements (two or three times a day is healthy and normal). If you are not assimilating and eliminating effectively, this not only affects your

weight, but other physical conditions as well. More fiber from food, herbs, and drinking more water all help with elimination. Be cautious of psyllium and other "binding" laxatives as they may only make you bloat or stop up. Consider Benefiber® instead.

Herbs

Garcinia – reduces appetite, increases energy

Chickweed – diuretic, digestive aid, lowers bowel transit time

Cascara Sagrada – good for chronic constipation, non-habit forming

Licorice – beneficial to all glands, do not take if you have high blood pressure

Kelp – natural source of vitamins and minerals

Aromatherapy

Geranium	Clary Sage	Cypress
Grapefruit	Lemon	Lime
Orange		

Visualization

Relax and take a breath. Picture and imagine a table before you containing many fattening foods, full of sugar, fat and calories. You know these are not good for you, so you sweep them off the table with one wave of your arm. Now picture a table before you with only good, healthy, nourishing foods that you love and know are good for your body, mind, and spirit. Choose a favorite food from this table. Then savor each bite as you chew it slowly and thoroughly. Breathe in, feel content, and satisfied.

AFFIRMATIONS

I deeply and completely love and accept myself right now.

I allow and encourage my body to transform calories into abundant energy.

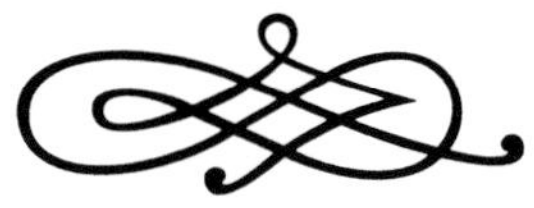

1. James F. Balch, M.D., Phyllis A. Balch, C.N.C., Prescription for Nutritional Healing, Avery Publishing Group, 1990, pg. 166.

2. Diane Stein, *The Natural Remedy Book for Women,* The Crossing Press, pg. 129.

3. Christiane Northrup, M.D., *Women's Bodies, Women's Wisdom,* Bantam Books, 1994, pg. 172.

4. Dr. Linda Page, *Healthy Healing Guide To Menopause & Osteoporosis,* Healthy Healing Publications, 1997, page 51.

5. Chistiane Northrup, M.D., *Health Secrets for Women,* Phillips Publishing, 1995, pg. 17.

6. Christiane Northrup, M.D., *Women's Bodies Women's Wisdom,* Bantam Books, New York, 1994, pg. 467.

7. Sally Fallon, M.A. & Mary Enig, Ph.D., "Butter is Better," *Health Freedom News,* Nov/Dec 1995.

8. Diane Stein, *The Natural Remedy Book for Women,* The Crossing Press, 1992, pg. 264.

9. *AARP Bulletin,* Feb. 27, Vol. 38 #2, 1997.

10. Weil, Andrew, "Reflexology Offers Whole-Body Benefits," *Self Healing Newsletter,* May, 1997.

11. Susun S. Weed, *Menopausal Years, The Wise Woman Way,* Ash Tree Publishing, New York, 1992, page 70.

12. Dr. Susan Love, *Hormone Book,* Random House, New York, 1997, pg. 55.

13. John R. Lee, M.D., *What Your Doctor May Not Tell You About Menopause,* Warner Books, New York, 1996, pg. 238.

– *Part III* –

Alternative Therapies

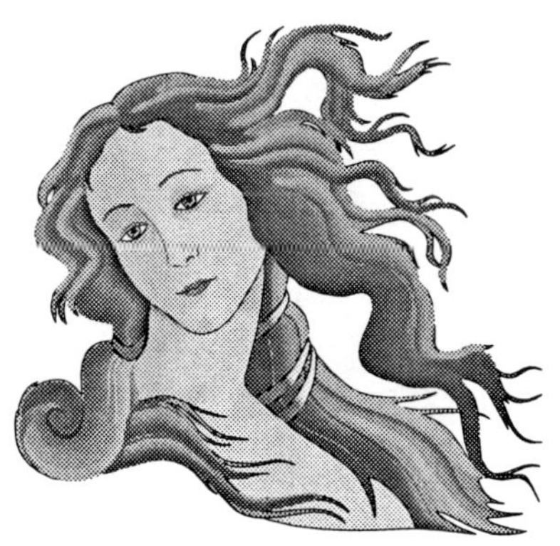

"The good news is that there are many natural remedies for the symptoms of menopause. I am so thrilled to find this book, and it is a great reference for me."

Susan G., Age 48
Career Coach and Consultant

Aromatherapy

Aromatherapy is a truly effective and magical way of influencing and healing the body, mind, and spirit. The term "Aromatherapy" was coined in the early 1920's in France, however, the practice of aromatherapy has been around for thousands of years. It has ancient roots as far back as Egypt, India, Persia and Europe, and even the Bible tells of the Wise Men who brought gifts of frankincense and myrrh to the baby Jesus.

Today, we think of aromatherapy as fragrances, however, it is much more. Scents affect us on many levels and elicit profound effects just through inhalation. For now, let me briefly describe aromatherapy and how you may use it for your own well-being and self-healing.

Aromatherapy is the use of aromatics or Essential Oils to promote healing of the body, mind, emotions, and spirit. Because Essential Oils are botanical, they harmonize well with the body. Essential Oils are the concentrated active ingredients of plants. These substances, to a greater or lesser degree, contain hormones, vitamins, antibiotics, and antiseptics. In addition, they are germicidal, antiviral, antidepressant, aphrodisiacs, hormonal balancers, detoxifiers, anticarcinogenic, mental stimulating, fever and blood pressure reducing, and much more.

Cautions And Guidelines:

Because they are so highly concentrated, **use Essential Oils by the drop only. do not take oils internally. Use with caution. Keep away from your eyes and from children. Check if you are sensitive to an oil by rubbing a drop on the inside of your elbow and waiting for an hour or so.**

Suggestions for using oils include:

Baths	Massage Oils	Perfumes
Diffusers	Compresses	Inhalers
Oils and Lotions	Shampoos	Soaps

My favorite remedy for so many things and which you see in this book is an **AROMATHERAPY BATH.** See description following this section.

True Essential Oils come in brown or blue bottles. Store them away from heat and light so they will not deteriorate. Prices differ based on the type of oil, how it is processed, and where it comes from.

The oils are so highly concentrated they will smell very strong in the bottles, however, when you dilute them in baths, lotions, oils, or sprays, you can appreciate their qualities much more.

Using Scents For Yourself

You can use Essential Oils in many different ways. As you begin to use them, you will learn more and more ways to enjoy them and discover which ones you prefer. After all, the ones that appeal to you are the ones that work best for you. Following are a few suggestions you might wish to try.

BATHS – Add six to eight drops to a bath under running water. Swish to mix the oil around in the water before you get in. Or you can add your favorite scent to a bubble bath or bath oil. Then, relax and enjoy.

CARRY SCENT WITH YOU – Put a drop on the corner of a handkerchief and carry it in your purse or pocket. Whenever you need a lift pull it out and take a whiff. Just opening your purse releases some of the delightful fragrance. Scents are used to relax, refresh, and stimulate. Try putting a drop of Essential Oil on a cotton ball and carrying that with you in a pocket as well.

RELEASE INTO THE AIR – Vaporizers, diffusers, scent balls, atomizers, candles, and light bulb rings are all ways to distribute a fragrance into the air. Scents have effects on anyone in a room where they are being used.

LOTIONS AND OILS – Make your own scented lotions or oils by using unscented bases and adding your own favorite fragrance. Use approximately ten to twenty drops of Essential Oil per two ounces of oil or lotion. Use pure oils and lotions with no mineral oil.

MASSAGE OIL ON FEET – Getting a massage is always wonderful. Essential Oils may be added to different massage or carrier oils, and indeed, some oils are sold this way. If you are not sensitive to an Essential Oil, you can massage it on your feet either by itself or mixed in a carrier oil.

Primary Women's Hormone Balancing Essential Oils are: GERANIUM, CLARY SAGE, AND LAVENDER.

A good place to rub Geranium, Clary Sage, or Lavender (for female concerns) is around the inside and outside of the ankles.

The Essential Oils

Following are oils that are mentioned in this book. Many oils have overlapping effects, so if you want to start with one oil, choose Lavender. If you are perimenopausal or menopausal, then choose Geranium or Clary Sage. However, always let your nose be your guide. In other words, whatever appeals to you will be the best one for you.

LAVENDER: The "universal" oil. One of the most balanced and safe oils, used for many types of skin conditions, especially helpful for burns. Safe to be used directly on skin, good for insomnia, anxiety, it's antiseptic, brings down high blood pressure, much more. When in doubt, use Lavender.

CHAMOMILE: Reduces any kind of inflammation, calms irritated skin, helpful for irregular periods, vaginitis, menopausal problems, PMS, diuretic properties, it's an anti-depressant, good for headaches, migraines, sedative action, stabilizes emotions, safe for children.

CEDARWOOD: Good for respiratory problems, promotes urination, useful against, urinary infections, prostrate problems, combats infection, cystitis, controls pain, fights fungal infections, calming, eases anxiety, stabilizes energy.

CLARY SAGE: Contains hormone-like components that can balance female hormones. Used to diminish menopausal symptoms, menstrual cramps, PMS, cool hot flashes, ease migraines, good for wrinkles, depression, and nerves.

CYPRESS: Stimulates circulation and has detoxifying effect on entire body. Relieves pain and muscle spasm, fights infection, constricts blood vessels, tightens tissues, inhibits bleeding, soothes upset emotions, gives support during major transitions.

EUCALYPTUS: Widely used in cold and flu remedies, clearing to the respiratory system, decongesting, loosens mucus, phlegm, enhances immune system, good for sore muscles, disinfecting, clearing, stimulating.

GERANIUM: An antidepressant with hormonal action, helpful for PMS, perimenopause, menopause, inflammation of the breast, aids lymphatic and circulatory system, helpful for fluid retention, broken capillaries, sore throats, wounds, and is very calming.

GRAPEFRUIT: Astringent to the skin. Helps drain lymphs, for water retention, obesity, cellulitis, good for digestive problems. Stimulating and anti-depressant. Used for menopausal problems, PMS, and hot flashes.

JASMINE: Eases labor pains, encourages contractions, fights infection, clears excess mucus, diminishes depression, calms nerves. Not to be used during pregnancy. (This is a more expensive oil to purchase).

JUNIPER: Used for centuries for urinary tract problems, eliminates wastes from body especially after too much rich food or alcohol, regulates menstrual cycle, reduces fluid retention, eases hemorrhoids, enlivens dull skin, clears acne, gives mental clarity.

LEMON: Lemon is antibacterial, cooling and refreshing. Helps fight infection, balances overactive oil glands, cools fever, lowers high blood pressure, tightens and tones tissues, promotes bowel movements, increases urination, eases fear, and calms.

MARJORAM: Lowers blood pressure, dilates blood vessels, improves circulation, helps with PMS, cramps, stimulates menstrual flow, relieves gas, upset stomach, headaches, speeds healing, good for insomnia, relieves tension.

PEPPERMINT: Stimulates the central nervous system, stimulates menstrual flow and eases the pain, relieves digestive problems, relaxes tense muscles, fights infection, clears congestion, regulates oiliness, cools emotions, dissipates anger and hysteria.

PINE: Fights infection, relieves muscle and joint pain, clears congestion and increases urination. Also, increases blood pressure and stimulates the adrenal glands. Restores strength after physical weakness or during convalescence.

ROSE: Balances female hormones, strengthens digestive system, helps overcome constipation, nausea, vomiting, good for migraines, headaches, soothes emotions, elevates spirits, can ease grief, gentle enough for children. (This is a more expensive oil to purchase and can cost into hundreds of dollars for one ounce.)

ROSEMARY: Stimulates circulation and raises low blood pressure. Excellent for toning entire body, boosting immune system, relieves digestive disorders, stimulates activities of internal organs, helps overcome mental fatigue, enhances mental alertness.

ROSEWOOD: Overall tonic for body, boosts immune system, deters colds, eases headache, reduces itching of psoriasis, eczema, helps with wrinkles, can diminish scars, relieves anxiety and stress, balances emotions.

SANDALWOOD: Stimulates immune system, fights infections such as cystitis, prostatitis, urethritis. It relieves diarrhea, earaches, respiratory infections, itching and skin complaints. It is mild on the skin and helps hydrate dry skin.

TEA TREE: Also known as Melaleuca has a broad spectrum of uses. It is antibacterial, antifungal, used for bites, blisters, burns, cuts, skin disorders, dandruff, colds, fevers, sore throats, increases immunity, helps restore energy.

YLANG YLANG: Lowers blood pressure, regulates respiration, eases muscle spasms, useful for irregular periods, cramps, PMS, calms through menopause years, soothes nerves, lifts depression, and has aphrodisiac effects.

OILS TO AVOID IF PREGNANT (may be harmful to fetus or cause miscarriage): Anise, Basil, Camphor, Cedarwood, Cinnamon, Clary Sage, Clove, Cypress, Eucalyptus, Fennel, Hyssop, Jasmine, Juniper, Marjoram, Mint, Myrrh, Oregano, Rosemary, Sage, Thyme, Wintergreen. (Avoid the oils, but not necessarily the food spices used in cooking; they are not the same).

Relaxing Aromatherapy Bath

One of the most delightful, restful and effective ways to de-stress and feel simply wonderful is to take a relaxing Aromatherapy Bath. Here's my personal recipe:

Start by filling a bathtub with warm water that is a temperature comfortable for you. Under the running water add:

- 1 cup Epsom Salts
- Favorite bubble bath
- 6 to 8 drops of you favorite Essential Oil or oils

Lavender, geranium and sandalwood are my favorites. Use a single oil or a couple different ones. Aromatherapy bath oils can also be purchased. One of my favorite ones to buy is Kneipp Herbal Baths (Spruce and Pine scent).

Next:

- Set out several candles in the bathroom and light them
- I prepare myself a cup of herbal tea (raspberry or chamomile) or a cup of hot water with lemon and honey
- Dim the lights or put on a night light, and of course the candles provide light too
- Turn on your favorite, soft music, or simply enjoy the silence
- Relax in the bath for about twenty minutes
- While you are in the bath, if you need healing or peace in some area of your life, imagine, picture, feel, or simply pray for that healing to occur in the best way. I know you will find this experience relaxing, refreshing and a delightful way to start or end any day.

  ENJOY!!!

Words Of Caution

When adding Essential Oils to the bath, be sure you "swish" them well in the water. A good idea is to mix the Essential Oils with a carrier oil such as almond or grape seed oil and then add that to the bath. Do not use oils that you may be allergic to or that contain mineral oil. Peppermint and citrus oils can be too strong for a bath unless well diluted. Again, some of the best oils to use for female conditions are Geranium, Clary Sage, or Lavender.

Calcium – Magnesium

Calcium is one of the most important minerals in your body, and it is essential to your bones, teeth, nerves, heart, muscles, metabolism, and much more. Calcium is needed to keep bones strong and help prevent osteoporosis. Magnesium is also an extremely important mineral and especially so, because without it, calcium cannot do it's job. They work together.

Sufficient magnesium is needed for better calcium absorption, and to help place it in the bones where it belongs. It is important to balance your diet with both calcium and magnesium. The standard American diet is low in magnesium. If a diet is low in magnesium and high in calcium (by comparison), this can actually contribute to osteoporosis.

Food is the best way to get both calcium and magnesium. However, getting enough of both can be a challenge, especially when so many things can deplete these minerals from the body such as stress. Keep in mind that it is a good idea to take a supplement.

Calcium Benefits – What It Can Do For You,

Prevent Osteoporosis
Relieve Muscle & Leg Cramps
Benefit Nerves & Nervousness
Prevent Headaches & Migraines
Needed for Blood Clotting
Preventative for Colon Cancer
Makes Strong Teeth & Bones
Aid Premenstrual Stress
Help Insomnia
Help Arthritis
Lower Cholesterol
Regulate Heartbeat

Magnesium Benefits – What It Can Do For You

A Must for Calcium Absorption
Aid for PMS Symptoms
Reduces Chocolate Cravings
Lowers Blood Pressure
Needed for Muscle Function
Helps Irregular Heartbeat
Prevent Kidney Stones & Gallstones
Relieves Migraines
Soothes Nerves
Increases Energy
Protects Artery Lining
Aid Mental Confusion

Supplementation needs vary based on your specific body type, lifestyle, and personal habits. Take calcium and magnesium in a ratio of at least 2:1; some suggest taking equal parts calcium to magnesium, i.e. 1:1. Food and supplements should both be considered when looking at your total calcium/magnesium intake. The following guidelines may be helpful when selecting a supplement.

1. If Perimenopausal – get at least 1000-1200 mg. of Calcium and 500-600mg. of Magnesium per day.
2. If Menopausal – you need 1500 mg. of Calcium and 800 mg. of Magnisium per day.

Not all supplements are created equal! Brands vary tremendously depending on the calcium source, the combination, and the amount. Some nutrients enhance calcium absorption and assimilation such as boron, zinc, manganese, silica. In addition, many herbs are high in calcium and are often easier to absorb.

Supplement Buying Guidelines

- Avoid all compounds containing bone meal, dolomite, and oyster shell. These are not absorbed well by the body, and the FDA cautions they may contain lead.
- **Calcium citrate** is one of the best and easiest to assimilate.
- **Microcrystalline Hydroxyapatite**, from whole bone extract, is also highly absorbable and has been shown in studies to stop bone loss and regenerate bone as well. If you already have osteoporosis, this is one to consider.
- **Check labels** for the amount, and buy combinations with a calcium *and* magnesium ratio of 2:1 or 1:1.
- Supplements containing boron are excellent as **boron** aids in calcium assimilation.
- Do not buy brands that contain sugar, flavoring, hydrogenated oils, artificial sweeteners, or other additives. I prefer capsules to tablets for easier swallowing and absorption.
- **Chelated brands** are sometimes easier for the body to absorb and utilize.

- Take calcium/magnesium supplements throughout the day in **smaller doses to enhance absorption**. For example, take one or two tablets in the morning, at mid-day and before bed (calcium helps you sleep and is absorbed better while sleeping).
- Avoid taking calcium with whole grains such as cereal or whole wheat bread. Some of the **calcium binds with the fiber** and does not get absorbed.
- Do not rely solely on dairy products to fulfill calcium needs (there is often too much calcium to magnesium). Look to a **balanced diet** that includes leafy greens, whole grains, fruits, nuts, etc. Variety is best.
- ***Daily* consumption of oxalic acid** found in cooked spinach, rhubarb, asparagus, and chocolate inhibits calcium absorption. Eat these in moderation.
- **Do not take Tums for calcium.** It's calcium carbonate which is not easily assimilated.
- **Herbs** are very high in calcium content as well, and are considered foods because they come from food. Try these: Barberry Bark, Horsetail, Kelp, Nettles, Oatstraw, Plaintain, White Oak Bark, and Valerian.

Items That Deplete Calcium

Certain foods, drugs and activities deplete or inhibit calcium activity in the body. Better to restrict or avoid the following:

- Carbonated Beverages (All sodas whether diet or not!)
- Alcohol
- Antacids and Aluminum
- Stress
- Chronic Dieting
- Cortisone, Prednisone, Steroid Drugs
- Caffeine
- Sugar
- Protein – especially red meat
- Smoking
- Lack of Exercise or Over-Exercise
- Fluoride or Fluoridated Water

Calcium & Magnesium Foods

Calcium and magnesium rich foods from natural, unprocessed sources are the best. Leafy green vegetables and grains are excellent sources for both. Dairy products are a good source of calcium but not for magnesium. When consuming dairy products, try certified raw dairy, which is superior in taste and in vitamin/mineral content, and it is easier to digest. In fact, some people can tolerate certified raw dairy when they cannot tolerate regular dairy! Certified raw is safe and tastes great. The drawbacks are that it costs a little more, and it does not have the shelf-life of regular dairy products.

Vitamin D and potassium are also important as are many other nutrients not covered in this section. The sun is your best source of Vitamin D. Sit or walk in the sun for five to ten minutes a day and you will get plenty of Vitamin D. Potassium is available in many of the foods listed here. Remember, eat a well-balanced diet and include many whole, natural, unprocessed, and organic foods whenever possible.

Good Calcium Choices Include:

Oatmeal, Tofu, Cheese (Parmesan, Cottage, Feta are good), Sesame Seeds, Yogurt, Figs, Molasses, Soy Nuts, Almonds, Salmon, Kale, Miso, Broccoli.

Good Magnesium Choices Include:

Wheatgerm, Sunflower Seeds, Figs, Soy Nuts, Almonds, Bananas, Eggs, Liver, Legumes, Broccoli, Millet, Miso, Black-eyed peas, Curry, Mustard Powder.

Castor Oil Packs

Castor Oil's healing and therapeutic values have been known and used for centuries. It is also known as Palma Christi meaning the "balm of Christ." Edgar Cayce, a well-known psychic, popularized the remedy in the 1940's, and in fact, some people claimed it was the miracle they were looking for.

Castor oil packs can be used for both internal or external conditions. It is helpful for female cramps, joint aches and pains, abdominal stress, and has been shown to improve the immune system as well. This method takes a little more time and trouble, but it is well worth it.

Castor oil can be rubbed directly on the skin for warts, arthritic joints, bruises, psoriasis, skin cancer, acne, boils, herpes, and more. When castor oil is applied externally for internal ailments it soothes and helps with breast lumps, uterine and ovarian cysts, tumors, gall bladder trouble, and liver problems. It aids in detoxification, in general.

Castor oil has an oily texture so be sure to protect your clothes and linens by wrapping the body part that needs attention in a wrap or bandage. You may purchase castor oil in most drug stores. Following is a recipe you can try. Good luck and enjoy!

How To Make A Castor Oil Pack

Use three to five times a week for about one hour until desired results are achieved.

1. Fold a washcloth, dishtowel, or piece of wool flannel, and soak it in warm castor oil until it is wet but not dripping.
2. Place saturated cloth directly over the body part that needs healing.
3. Cover the pack with a plastic bag, a wrap, or a plastic sheet to protect linen and garments.
4. Place heating pad or, preferably a hot water bottle or other non-electrical heating source, over everything.
5. Wrap a towel around everything.

6. Relax for up to an hour or more while you mentally send healing energy to the area.

When Finished

Remove pack and wash skin with a solution of water and baking soda (about two teaspoons to a quart of water) to remove castor oil and any secretions from skin. The pack may be stored in a plastic bag and re-used. Just add additional oil as necessary.

Exercise

A new study released on April 23, 1997, by the *Journal of the American Medical Association (JAMA)*, reports that exercise is *as effective* in prolonging life for post-menopausal women as taking estrogen replacement, and it's *safer!* Statistics indicate that exercising even once a week decreases death rate by twenty-four percent, exercising two to four times a week by thirty percent, and exercising four or more times per week by thirty-eight percent. This is especially effective in reducing death rate due to heart disease!

Exercise is, by far, the best thing you can do for yourself, no matter what your age or your potential risk condition. For perimenopause and menopause, incorporate some weight-bearing exercise along with anything else you might do (see section on "Osteoporosis"). What else can exercise do for you?

- Improves circulation throughout the entire body
- Increases muscle strength and tones muscles
- Makes bones stronger, especially if it is a weight-bearing exercise
- Helps burn fat, so keeps weight in check
- Lowers blood pressure and resting heart rate
- Strengthens heart function
- Raises HDL (the good cholesterol)
- Helps move out toxins from the tissues
- Increases endorphins which are the body's natural opiates and antidepressants
- Reduces stress
- Improves moods
- Enhances posture

Studies have shown that exercise, in and of itself, assists with many physical problems and conditions. It can also:

- Reduce hot flashes
- Reverse bone loss
- Increase bone mass
- Improve elimination
- Reduce heart disease risk
- Relieve tension and anxiety
- Relax and aid sleep
- Increase self-esteem

Finding Your Own Special Exercise

The key is to find an exercise or sport that you *like,* and then *do it!* If you hate jogging, don't take it up. If all you want to do is floor exercises in front of the television, *do it!* At least start that way and then work up to something more challenging. Start with a small commitment (it's easier to keep). For example, commit to five minutes a day of something! When you've done that for several weeks, you'll be ready and willing to move forward to something else. One of the things I enjoy is working out at Curves For Women®. They offer a thirty-minute fitness workout and have locations all over the country.

Easy Exercise Ideas

- Take the stairs instead of the elevator.
- Walk your dog and let him take you for a run.
- Try out a gym or, better yet, check out Curves For Women® in your area.
- Buy a mini-trampoline. It's great for weight-bearing exercise, easy on the joints, good for circulation, and can be done at home.
- Go swimming.
- Jump rope.
- Take a yoga class, dance class, or self-defense class.
- Buy an easy exercise tape (how about Richard Simmons)!
- Take tennis lessons or take up volleyball, baseball, or some other sport of your choice.
- Just stretch every morning and breathe deeply throughout the day.

Walking – The Best

Walking is the best and easiest exercise you can do. No special equipment or clothes are needed. All you need is comfortable shoes. You can do it anytime of day, on your lunch break, or after dinner. It's free, it's healthy, and it's weight-bearing.

Weight-bearing exercise helps build and preserve the bones. Walking is good for the heart because it provides circulation to the whole body, and it lifts your spirits. Many people say they look forward to their walk and wonder how they ever did without it. Take a walk outside in nature. Feel the earth beneath your feet, smell the fresh air, and admire Mother Nature and all Her beauty. You can start a walking program by walking just ten or twenty minutes a day. When you feel ready, work up to more time and more distance over several weeks or months. I like to walk in the mornings when it's cool and the dew is still on the grass. It's a magical time of day!

Yoga – Another Easy Exercise

A few good words about yoga. It is an all-around practice that anyone can do plus gain benefits. It is an ancient exercise regime developed thousands of years ago by Eastern sages. There are several different types of yoga, but in general it offers physical, mental, and spiritual conditioning, and is considered a meditation by many. In yoga, you do asanas or postures which consist of breathing and stretching. *Breathing* is integral to yoga. Yoga relaxes the body, improves circulation, and adds flexibility, and clears the mind.

Yoga has become much more popular in recent years. It is a practice that improves energy and claims to slow down the aging process! You can buy tapes and practice it at home, or check into classes in your area.

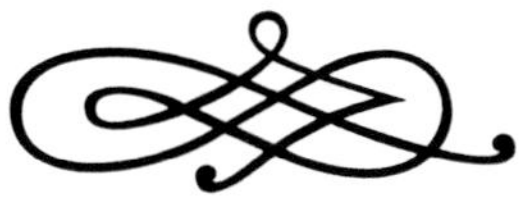

Herbs

Herbs are God's gift to man from Mother Earth. In the Apocrypha, Ecclesiastes, 34, 4 it says, "The Lord hath created medicines out of the earth, and he that is wise will not abhor them." Herbs have been around for thousands of years and are used regularly, even today. Every other culture in the world uses them, except America. Before drugs, we had herbs. Why use herbs? Herbs are used to maintain good health, to correct or help correct numerous health problems through elimination and detoxification, to build and strengthen the body and its organs, to improve health in general, to rebuild the body following an illness or trauma, to aid in weight loss and weight control, and to assist in many specific conditions from acne to PMS to menopause.

Differences Between Herbs And Drugs

HERBS	DRUGS
Come from Nature, such as plants, trees, roots, flowers, etc. Herbs are food.	Synthetically manufactured in a lab or from animal sources. (Although many "isolated" synthetics originally came from Nature.)
Gentle – in harmony with the body because they are botanical. Side "benefits" that assist other conditions in the body in addition to the reason you are taking it.	Stronger – more harsh and have side effects which can be damaging to the body or other organs.
Contain natural buffers because they come from the whole plant.	Active ingredients are isolated out to create a specific effect on a particular symptom or problem in the body.
Herbs take longer to work sometimes. Take for several weeks or months to achieve best results.	Rapid, immediate results and strong effect.

HERBS	DRUGS
No withdrawal and effects may be permanent after consistently taking an herb over a period of time.	Drugs address the "symptom" and rarely the cause. Withdrawal may create more problems and you still have the same condition.
Nature is man's best friend!	Nothing "man-made" can compete or duplicate what Mother Nature can do!
Contain vitamins and minerals.	Can interfere with absorption of vitamins and minerals (supplements or foods).

Herbs are extremely beneficial and effective with many women's conditions. Following are twelve significant herbs used successfully with many women's conditions. There are many more herbs than can be discussed here. I encourage you to read more about herbs. A couple excellent books are *The Way of Herbs* by Michael Tierra, C.H., N.D. and *Earl Mindell's Herb Bible* by Earl Mindell, R.Ph, Ph.D. Easy and fun to read along with much good information.

When purchasing herbs remember **all herbs are not created equal.** They differ in quality and strength from brand to brand. A good herbalist, holistic health practitioner, some chiropractors, and others educated in this area can often advise you on the best brands to purchase. Health food stores and some drug stores carry good brands. Generic brands can vary in quality because, unless someone knows the product, there is no way to know the quality. Price is not always an indicator of the best, so ask questions. In the end, the best determination of quality is the effect it has on you! Remember, give herbs a fair chance and some time to work in your body.

Ways To Take Herbs

You can take herbs in several different ways. They can be purchased as **capsules, tablets, tinctures, teas, or as dry herbs.** Personally, I like to use capsules because they work well for me. They are easy to swallow and are easy to digest. Compressed tablets are harder to digest. Tinctures are great because they are liquid. Liquids are easier to absorb and get into your blood stream more quickly. Be aware that tinctures are usually in an alcohol base, and this may or may not be a satisfactory method for some people. You can at times get some tinctures in glycerine (tastes sweet and has no alcohol).

Teas are excellent, and may be a good way to start for some people. They can be used simply as a drink, and as such, are very helpful for many conditions. Green tea, for example, is a great substitute for coffee. Like coffee, it has caffeine, however it is not the same kind of caffeine. It has many other beneficial effects such as being anti-cancer, anti-tumor, anti-oxidant, lowers cholesterol, lowers blood pressure, protects from carcinogens, and is naturally cooling to the body.

Teas can be used therapeutically. To use therapeutically means the final tea is much stronger than regular sipping tea. For example, regular chamomile tea makes a nice drink and can be quite helpful for many people. For a more therapeutic use, steep the tea with three or more tea bags. It will taste very strong. Dry herbs are great for making your own teas and tinctures as well. However, this is time consuming and messy so most people don't have the time or patience to do it.

My suggestion would be to **try tinctures, capsules next,** and drink the **herb teas** in place of coffee or caffeinated teas.

Herbs For Women

BLACK COHOSH has estrogenic properties, which means it can take the place of estrogen in the body. It can help regulate estrogen, reduce hot flashes, calm the nervous system, help insomnia, support kidneys and liver, and increase digestive juices. This is one of the herbs that can help support you through menopause, especially if you experience hot flashes. It is best not take this for longer than six months, especially if taking it alone. However, it seems to work best in combination with other herb products. Remifemin®, which comes from Germany, is available in many stores and its primary ingredient is Black Cohosh.

BLUE COHOSH is another herb often used for menstrual irregularities, amenorrhea (lack of menses), and dysmenorrhea (painful menstruation). Though not related to Black Cohosh, they have similar properties. It acts as an antispasmodic and can be used before or during actual childbirth as well.

DONG QUAI is an Eastern herb used to correct many female problems. This is helpful for hot flashes, regulating menses, relieving uterine pain, adding moisture to vaginal tissues, reducing headaches, helping with water retention, heart palpitations, insomnia, restoring youth to skin, and toning liver. This is not recommended if experiencing heavy bleeding. Dong Quai is often found in Chinese tea remedies for female problems.

GINSENG has been found to be very helpful for hot flashes. It is a stimulant and an adaptogen, which means it helps the body adapt to stress and changes. Excellent herb for stress and fatigue. Ginseng also helps to normalize the body processes and has a reputation for reducing cholesterol and inhibiting growth of cancerous tumors.

MOTHERWORT is a good heart tonic, reduces palpitations, promotes circulation, and helps angina. It also relieves PMS, menstrual cramps, constipation, hot flashes, eases stressed nerves, depression, relieves anxiety, helps with insomnia, and restores elasticity to the vaginal walls.

NETTLES is an important bitter herb which is helpful for urinary inflammations including cystitis and nephritis. It halts excessive bleeding, improves weakness, and is good for hemorrhoids, chronic arthritis, and rheumatic conditions.

RED CLOVER contains isoflavones and is part of the group of phytoestrogens. It has long been used as a blood purifier, which means it supports liver function, is good for skin eruptions, psoriasis, and mucus congestion. It is helpful for reducing or shrinking tumors, and is often recommended as a supplement if you have cancer.

SAGE helps eliminate night sweats, hot flashes, regulates hormones, calms nerves, helpful for depression, headaches, digestion, cramps, bladder infections, joint aches, mental clarity, improves circulation, and relieves dizziness.

ST. JOHN'S WORT has been found to be a good alternative to antidepressant drugs. It is a sedative and an antidepressant.

This is good for depression, nervousness, anxiety, muscle and joint pains. People with minor depression, who have taken Prozac in the past, often experience positive results with this herb. It is better to take one or the other, but not both.

VALERIAN has a sedative action and is excellent for inducing a restful sleep. Unlike sleeping drugs, valerian allows you get a good night's sleep and awaken refreshed. It is often used as a nerve tonic, for headaches, muscle spasms, and cramps. Valerian has a strong, rather unpleasant smell, yet don't let that deter you. It really works!

VITEX also known as CHASTE TREE is very helpful in normalizing the menstrual cycle, and increases progesterone and estrogen. It is an excellent female herb and must be taken over a period of time (as much as three to six months) before its affects are truly appreciated. Vitex is effective in relieving symptoms of PMS as well as reducing hot flashes, fibroids, dizziness, endometriosis, constipation, digestion, skin disorders, and more.

WILD YAM contains hormone precursors called diosgenin. It is used to make natural progesterone found in progesterone creams. It can also be taken internally and is very helpful for cramps, for improving liver and gallbladder function. It is helpful for many of the problems connected with low progesterone levels.

There are many, many more herbs that are effective and helpful. *Some* of them are:

ALFALFA – nutritive, supports pituitary, whole body, and liver.

BLESSED THISTLE – for stomach and liver, relieves fevers, and bleeding.

BURDOCK – a blood purifier especially for arthritis and acne.

CAYENNE – for circulation and used as catalyst for other herbs, stops bleeding internally and externally.

CASCARA SAGRADA – an aid for constipation and gall stones.

CHICKWEED – assists cholesterol problems and assists in weight loss.

CORNSILK – aids painful urination, and supports kidneys and bladder.

CRANBERRY – helps with cystitis, urinary and bladder problems.

ECHINACEA – a natural antibiotic which enhances the immune system and supports the lymph glands.

GARLIC – emulsifies cholesterol, helps reduce infections, and is an immune builder.

GOLDENSEAL – like a natural antibiotic and helps support liver.

HAWTHORN – heart tonic, high in magnesium and supports blood vessels.

KELP – effective in supporting thyroid and arteries.

LICORICE ROOT – balances blood sugar and supports adrenal glands.

PARSLEY – high in Vitamin B and Potassium.

PASSION FLOWER – sedative, good for sore muscles, headaches, neuralgia.

PAU D'ARCO – blood builder and discourages growth of candida.

RED RASPBERRY – uterine toner for women at all ages and helps relieve cramps.

SARSAPARILLA – similar to the male hormone testosterone so can assist with libido. It is also good for gout, psoriasis, rheumatism.

SHARK CARTILAGE – anti-cancer.

UVA URSI – for hemorrhoids, supports kidneys, spleen, liver, pancreas.

Massage

Massage is one of the healthiest remedies you can experience. It's even better for you if you are anxious, stressed, or feeling pain anywhere in your body. Hands-on therapy alleviates many physical and emotional conditions, and in addition, it is a preventative. Massage offers relaxation at the hands of a trained massage technician. Since all people are unique individuals, every person who practices massage will be different. They will be different even if they are doing the same type of massage. One of the most important things to know is that the experience of human touch is very healing.

Massage is beneficial to the body for almost anything and especially for stress. Stress is a major problem in our society and a contributing factor to most physical problems and illnesses. Everyone can benefit from a regular massage. Some of the benefits of massage include:

- Improves circulation to all areas of the body
- Stimulates lymph flow and detoxification
- Promotes relaxation
- Boosts immune system
- Increases energy and overall health
- Brings oxygen and nutrients to the tissues
- Provides positive experience of touch
- Helps to connect the body with the emotions

There are many different types of massage and far too many to mention here. However, most technicians offer a standard Swedish massage, which is designed for relaxation and destressing. It is a full body massage that you can request just about anywhere.

You may also hear about or wish to experience Reflexology. Reflexology is foot massage, which sometimes includes the hands too. It can be gentle or deep, depending on the practitioner or your desire. Reflexology works with pressure points on the feet and hands. It is a wonderful treatment and can be as fulfilling as a full body massage because the feet contain "reflex" points for the entire body, the organs, and muscles. (See section on "Reflexology").

Massage enhances healing at all levels, physical, mental, and emotional. If you do nothing else, treat yourself to a massage. It is still one of the least utilized and one of the most enjoyable and beneficial things you can do for yourself. Many chiropractors and clinics now offer massage. Sometimes, it's even covered by insurance, however, don't count on it. Hopefully, this is the future trend.

You may wish to try several different kinds of massage to find out which one you like best. There are other forms of massage besides Swedish, such as shiatsu or deep tissue, to mention a couple. Remember, everyone is different, so even the same kind of massage with a different therapist may feel different. Most are doing the best they know how in the way they were trained. Remember, you can always ask for lighter or deeper pressure, or extra work where you may need it. Thank them, be grateful, and your body will be grateful too. It's a good idea to leave a tip as well.

Give yourself the gift of massage today!

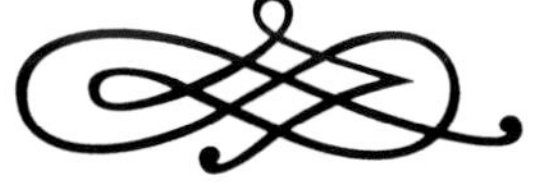

Nutrition

Good nutrition from food offers the basic ingredient to a healthy, disease free existence. With our hectic lifestyle, our desire for fast food and fast living, long work hours, stress, and overall lack of energy, it's very hard to eat a healthy optimal diet on daily basis. Please know that fatigue, stress, and many women's conditions can be alleviated by eating a healthy, nutritionally rich diet.

It is impossible to even begin to cover this issue adequately here. Nonetheless, a few basic guidelines are useful to almost any nutrition plan. There is no single diet or eating plan that works for everyone. What you must do is begin to find out what foods work for you, what foods don't work for you, and of the foods you like, which ones are healthy for you. This involves paying attention to your body, and knowing how it reacts when you eat certain foods.

You can start by noticing which foods energize you or which foods give a surge of energy and then deplete you. These are foods such as sugar, caffeine, and alcohol. It's also good to know which foods are your comfort foods, for example, ice cream and/or chocolate are often comfort foods. Knowing this can help you distinguish if you are eating out of physical or emotional hunger, or at least be able to make a choice.

Once again, it is up to you to become more informed by reading books, articles, and asking pertinent questions. Keeping a diary of the food you eat on a daily basis and writing down how you feel is a good way to start making connections between your emotions and the food you eat. Once you know this, you will be able to make wiser choices. You want to make choices that offer sustained energy as well as vitamins and minerals. Eating a healthy, nutritionally rich diet does not mean you can't enjoy your favorite chocolate pie. It simply means you'll enjoy it more because you will choose to eat it out of conscious choice for enjoyment and not out of some kind of emotional need.

Learn to dine. I believe if we were to really make our meals a dining experience, we would enjoy our food more. The more we enjoy food and the slower we eat, the more we actually taste our food. In that case, the happier and healthier our whole body will be. At home, try setting out flowers or candles with dinner, put on a tablecloth, or play some soothing music. Do not eat in front of the television, while going through the mail, and not while driving in traffic. Your body attempts to digest the entire experience of how and where you are eating, so make it a pleasant experience. You can do this for yourself and for your whole family. Why not make eating a time to communicate and share each other's company at least once a day.

Happy eating as you begin your nutritional journey!

Guidelines To Healthy Eating

- Eat OPTIMAL FOOD which is raw, fresh, whole, organic, and minimally processed foods eighty percent of the time.
- Eat less processed foods, sugar, caffeine, and alcohol.
- Eliminate margarine and all other hydrogenated fats and oils as best you can (a challenge considering many packaged foods contain hydrogenated oils, so read labels).
- Butter is healthy and better for you than margarine, yet eat in moderation.
- Eliminate all artificial sweeteners that contain aspartame. These affect the neurotransmitters in the brain and may cause side effects, such as headaches or dizziness. In addition, there's no proof they actually help you lose weight, and there's no nutritional benefit.
- Eat more fresh vegetables and fruits, especially in season. Organic produce has been proven to contain more natural vitamins and minerals than non-organic. If you are challenged in getting the appropriate servings of fruits and vegetables daily, try adding JuicePlus+® capsules (see "Resources" section.)
- Fresh is better than frozen. Frozen is better than canned.
- Eat less red meat.
- Reduce or eliminate processed bacon, hot-dogs, sandwich meats, etc.

- Avoid block type cheeses. These are real artery cloggers.
- Eat more complex carbohydrates (like brown rice, oatmeal, sweet potatoes, beans, lentils, etc.).
- Choose whole grains over white or wheat flour breads and pastas (rye and pumpernickel are also good).
- Drink eight 8 oz. glasses of water daily.
- Eliminate all carbonated beverages, except as an occasional treat. Carbonated drinks leach calcium from bones. Children should only drink these occasionally as well.
- Limit liquid intake to about four ounces (about one-half cup) with meals, otherwise liquids dilute digestive juices and inhibit absorption.
- Include one tablespoon of ground flax seeds daily, over cereals, salads, etc.
- Never take antacids, especially ones with aluminum. Most people need more digestive enzymes, not an antacid which inhibits the digestive juices. Try papaya and peppermint teas or mints instead.
- Stop eating at least three hours before retiring.
- Use common sense before embarking on any new diet program.
- CHEW, CHEW, CHEW, CHEW and most of your digestive problems will disappear and you will begin to really taste your food again. An old proverb says to *"Drink your food and chew your liquids."*

Please refer to other sections in the book for information on special conditions. As always, if in pain or seriously ill, be sure to consult your doctor or professional health care provider for further guidance.

Phytoestrogens

Phytoestrogens are a name for a group of nutrients derived from plants which have estrogen-like activities. They are considered weaker than our own body's estrogens. This means that the components of the phytoestrogens have both estrogenic and anti-estrogenic activities. Like estrogen, phytoestrogens compete for the same receptors in the body. Thus, phytoestrogens have been successful in helping decrease the symptoms of estrogen excess. These activities are related to the isoflavones or, as you may have heard them called, isoflavanoids.

Isoflavones are one of the main components of phytoestrogens. Recent studies report that isoflavones have very positive effects, including the following:

- Reduces risk of breast cancer.
- Reduces risk of other cancers including colon, lung, skin, prostrate.
- Reduces risk of atherosclerosis and related artery or coronary heart disease.
- Reduces LDL cholesterol (the "bad" cholesterol).
- Reduces risk of gall stones.
- Reduces inflammation and inflammatory pain.
- Stimulates new bone formation and offers bone-retaining properties.
- Provides relief from menopause symptoms such as hot flashes.

As you can see, phytoestrogens have many important properties in regard to women's conditions as well as other conditions, including lowering of blood pressure, offering resistance to osteoporosis, protection against symptoms of excess or dominant estrogen, and protection against many cancers including breast cancer.

Isoflavones are found in: **Alfalfa, apples, carrots, garbanzo beans, garlic, green beans, peas, barley, oats, red clover, and**

rye. They are also found in soy products. In fact, theories abound that perhaps it is the phytoestrogen-rich diet of Asian women that prevents them from experiencing the type of menopausal problems that American women experience. It is interesting to note that Japan has the lowest rate of breast and prostrate cancer in the world, however, also keep in mind that Japan eats a very low-fat diet in comparison to the high-fat diet of Americans.

Let's look at the soybean since it's been receiving lots of attention lately. **Soybeans are a good protein substitute,** and how they are processed and eaten is important. Soybeans are now used to mimic meat (soy burgers and soy dogs) and used as a substitute for dairy (soy milk). Be careful. Many of these products come from "isolated" soy protein which leave behind the other important nutrients of the whole soybean. For some people, soy is harder to digest, and may cause gastric upset and, as with anything, there can be allergic reactions.

It is the isoflavones or isoflavanoids you want and need. From the soy family they are found in roasted soy nuts, tofu, miso, soy milk, soy powder, tempeh, to name a few. They are not found, however, in plain soy sauce, soy formulas and drinks, soy oil, soy cheese, soy meats, or soy-protein concentrate foods such as soy burgers.

You must look for **whole soybean products** and *not* soybean isolate. You will notice there are many products containing soy isolates on the grocery shelf that you may already be eating, however, they are isolates and not that helpful for improving women's health symptoms or reducing the risk of cancer.

Fermented products are the easiest to digest, and my favorite is miso. Here's some soy products you may wish to try.

- **Miso** – Fermented soy paste, comes in red and white miso purchased from the refrigerated section. I do not recommend the dry mixes. Miso can be used as a soup itself and is full of minerals. Added to soups, it enhances flavor, or it can be used as a base for salad dressings and other sauces. Very tasty!
- **Tofu** – High protein custard or cheese-like cake. Comes in three main types: firm, soft, and silken. Firm works well in

recipes where density and shape are important, and silken tofu works well in products that are pureed or blended. A very versatile product that absorbs the taste and flavoring of foods with which it is blended. Note that tofu can be hard to digest for some.

- **Roasted Soy Nuts** – looks just like soy beans only roasted and salted. Great as a snack!
- **Soy Flour** – can be used in baked products that are not yeast-raised. Need to mix with other flour when baking.
- **Soy Powder** – found in protein drinks.
- **Tempeh** – Whole, cooked soybeans like a chewy cake, often used in place of meat.
- **Edamame** – Tender, young soybeans, salted, and cooked until tender. Sold in pods, shelled, canned or frozen.

Remember, isoflavones are also found in other vegetables, fruits and whole grains. "An apple a day" is still good nutritional advice, find organic, or at least unwaxed brands.

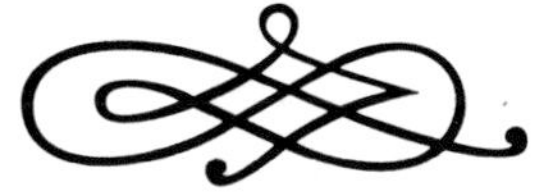

Progesterone Creams

Progesterone is the forgotten hormone. Plenty is written and heard about estrogen but what about progesterone? It is, at least, as important as estrogen. In addition, progesterone has the potential to revolutionize women's healthcare because it is so beneficial for many women's health conditions including PMS, perimenopause, menopause, and other hormonal imbalances. The key is that it must be ***natural* progesterone,** not progestin found in most pharmaceutical products.

Progestin is the synthetic form of progesterone, and it has many side effects (see section on "Hormone Replacement and Estrogen Replacement Therapy"). Though some people use these terms interchangeably, do not confuse them. If your doctor talks about progesterone, be sure to find out if he means progestin or natural progesterone. Natural progesterone is derived from soy products or wild yams, and it is safe, effective, and has **no side effects.**

As estrogen diminishes prior to and during perimenopause and menopause, so does progesterone, yet only more so. In fact, progesterone often diminishes long before you get to menopause and can start even when you are a young woman. This depends on your diet and lifestyle. These two hormones work synergistically to create a balance in your body, so if there is not enough progesterone in relation to estrogen, you get what's termed "estrogen dominance" or "excess estrogen." Too much estrogen plays a key role in almost all women's health conditions. It stands to reason that one good way to correct the imbalance is to add progesterone, not estrogen.

John R. Lee, M.D. is a doctor who is actively spreading the word about natural progesterone. Research exists showing that natural progesterone is beneficial for both osteoporosis and breast cancer, as well as many other female complaints. The best text to read for more detailed information on progesterone and what it can do for you is *What Your Doctor May Not Tell You About Menopause* by John R. Lee, M.D.

Functions of progesterone in the body include the following:

- Precursor of other sex hormones including estrogen!
- Protects against fibrocystic breasts
- Necessary during pregnancy
- Maintains uterine lining
- Natural diuretic
- Uses fat for energy
- Aids thyroid function
- Natural antidepressant
- Normalizes blood clotting
- Restores sex drive
- Helps normalize blood sugar levels
- Restores oxygen to cells
- Protects against endometrial and breast cancer
- Builds bone and is protective against osteoporosis

Progesterone creams can be one of the best remedies for many perimenopausal and menopausal symptoms as well as PMS. Progesterone has actually been around for quite awhile. It was primarily found in cosmetic creams, although there was not enough in those creams for therapeutic purposes discussed here. It is extremely important for you to know about progesterone creams. You want to know what they can do for you, and which ones to choose. Progesterone creams are not all the same.

Common Questions

What is Progesterone Cream?

It is a cream rubbed into the skin. It a natural product with an active ingredient called diosgenin that comes from wild yams or sometimes soy products. The natural progesterone appears "identical" to progesterone in the body and is, therefore, not synthetic. There have been no reported side effects and, in fact, it has many benefits. It is safe, easy to use, and can be purchased without a prescription.

Why a cream?

Progesterone is effectively delivered into the body transdermally, that is via the skin through the fat cells and released into the blood. This is the best way to take progesterone. Progesterone taken orally is broken down by the liver and once metabolized, little then remains available to the body.

How much should I use?

A non-pregnant, ovulating woman makes approximately twenty to twenty-four milligrams per day of progesterone for about twelve to fourteen days prior to her period, or about 240 milligrams per month. The amount absorbed from creams varies from woman to woman. Generally, it is recommended to use from 1/8 to 1/2 teaspoon of the cream, two times a day , for fourteen days before your period. The directions vary somewhat depending on if you are perimenopausal, menopausal, postmenopausal, or have PMS. Check the directions that come with the cream. In order to get adequate progesterone, be sure to purchase a cream with a minimum of 400 milligrams of progesterone per ounce.

Will I notice results right away?

You must use progesterone cream for at least three months to experience best results, however, you may very well experience results the first month. If you have been deficient in progesterone for several years, it may take a little longer to notice best results, or on the other hand, you may notice results immediately because your body is so deficient. Make a decision to use the cream regularly for at least three months, and take note of how your body feels.

Where do I apply the cream?

For better absorption, apply the cream on areas of the body that have thinner skin such as the chest, lower abdomen, inner thighs, wrists, back of hands, inner arms, and neck. Rotate the area where you rub in the cream in order to enhance absorption level.

Where can I buy progesterone cream?

Creams may be purchased without a prescription in many health product stores, some drug stores, and health food stores. You can also get the cream through holistic clinics or practitioners, who carry the cream and use it in their practice. Be sure to ask them how much progesterone is in the product. Check stores in your area to find out what kind of creams they carry. If they don't carry the brand you want, you might try asking them, and many will order it for you.

What kind should I buy?

All creams are not the same, however, creams usually come in two ounce jars or in tubes. Creams with a minimum of 800 milligrams of progesterone per two ounce jar are recommended. You may find creams in the marketplace which do not contain enough progesterone to make them worthwhile. For best results, use a cream that contains 400 milligrams or more per ounce. I use a proprietary blend of progesterone cream available to health care practitioners. I've also used Prolief by Arbonne International and had excellent results with both. For other brands, see the "Resources" section of this book, or look at the lists found in Dr. John Lee's or Dr. Susan Love's book mentioned below. Be aware there are creams that contain a combination of estrogen (often in a form called estriol) as well as progesterone. These creams are different and may have different effects. If you need additional estrogen, this is a safe way to get it. Be specific when asking for a cream and what would work best for you. For example, I recommend and sell the proprietary brand which contains natural progesterone and estriol. Arbonne International has a cream called PhytoProlief which contains natural progesterone, natural estrogen, and herbs. Make it a point to know what you are buying!

Will the amount of progesterone be listed on the jar?

No, not always! It is good to know what you are buying. A list of creams and progesterone amounts are found in Dr. John Lee's book *What Your Doctor May Not Tell You About Menopause* and in Dr. Susan Love's *Hormone Book.* The salespeople in the stores may not know the answer. Some creams contain only two to ten milligrams of progesterone, not nearly enough to be effective. However, some creams contain other ingredients such as herbs or oils that may be have benefit even though they don't contain the recommended amount of progesterone. These usually need to be tried in order to determine if they are helpful for you. If you wish to try the creams with herbs, try several of them, and then you can compare it to a progesterone cream that does contain the recommended amount of progesterone.

One reason you do not hear much about natural progesterone creams is because natural progesterone cannot be patented by a pharmaceutical company. Natural progesterone comes from natural substances, such as wild yams or soy products and therefore is not available for patent. Subsequently, it is not, as a rule, prescribed by doctors because they may not be aware of it, or because it's harder to know or regulate per individual how much is being absorbed through the skin. There are some knowledgeable doctors, however, who can write a prescription for natural hormones which can be purchased through a compounding pharmacy (see "Resources" section).

Give progesterone creams at least three consecutive months of use to experience best results. You may wish to keep a record of results for yourself and/or for your doctor. Progesterone is good for so many things including weight, moods, depression, fibrocystic breasts, hot flashes, as a preventative for breast and endometrial cancer as well as encouraging bone regeneration. Remember, the one that works for you is the best one.

Reflexology

Reflexology, in the simplest terms, is a delicious foot rub. It is the art and science of working with reflex points on the feet and/or hands. It has been around, at least, since ancient Egypt where paintings show people massaging each other's feet. In the early twentieth century, Reflexology was "rediscovered" by an American Dr. William Fitzgerald, and then taken up by Eunice Ingham, a massage therapist, who eventually created a map of the feet. The map indicates points of the body as reflected on the feet.

Reflexologists believe that certain reflex points on the feet are directly related to the body's organs, glands, and muscles, and by applying pressure to these points, many conditions, symptoms, aches and pains can be helped. Reflexology is known to relieve stress and tension, improve blood flow to certain areas, and assist in bringing relaxation and balance to the entire body. Just how this works, no one really knows, however, it may be related to the nerves and nervous system. In any case, it's well worth the experience.

If possible, find a trained Reflexologist. Some massage people are also trained in Reflexology and they may do a foot treatment that is similar and offers similar benefits. Persons associated with the International Institute of Reflexology or the North American Association of Reflexology should have enough training to provide a valuable service. However, do not rule out others you may find that you like and who know what they are doing.

Reflexology can be done every day. You may notice some tender or sensitive spots as your foot is being worked on. Pay attention to these spots and give them a little extra attention. By working these spots, signals are sent to the corresponding body part to relax and receive more circulation.

You can also work on your own feet. Here's some suggestions:

- Use a golf ball and roll the bottom of each foot on it.
- Put two or three golf balls in a sock and roll your feet over it.

- Try stretching your toes and circling your ankles to improve circulation.
- Do your own foot treatment by pressing between the toes and across the soles and tops of your feet. Apply pressure to tender spots for several minutes. The amount of pressure you use depends on the sensitivity of your feet. Do anything you like to loosen up your hands and feet.

Look for books on Reflexology in your local bookstore and library. There are many good ones from which to choose.

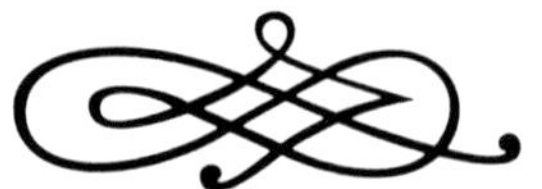

Relaxation Techniques

Relaxation is one of the most essential ingredients to achieve results with any health concern. You can achieve relaxation in many different ways. A few ideas have already been suggested throughout this guide. A little more detailed explanation is provided here for your convenience. When your body and mind are receptive and relaxed, you experience more healing benefits. Relaxation is so important because it reduces stress and brings peace to the body as well as the mind.

Relaxation can be found through breathing, meditation, visualization, affirmations, massage, hypnotherapy, prayer, listening to music, and much more. Exercise can relax the body and help relieve stress as well. You have many choices. People may prefer one or two techniques over others, but, I always say, "Whatever you like and will do, is what works best for you." So if you don't know, find out what you like. Try them all. Once you discover what you like and will do, then do it regularly!

All techniques are beneficial. Your intention is everything. What is your intention when you breathe or meditate or exercise? It's good to know what you want because then you will recognize it when it happens. For example, if your intention is to relax, you will. If your intention is to reduce pain, you will. If your intention is to boost your immune system, you will.

Now is your chance to choose which road to follow to achieve your desire.

AFFIRMATIONS are statements made over and over to encourage a desire, a healing, or a wish. Your belief in the result is very, very important. Make them positive and in the present tense. Many affirmations are presented in this guide, so now you can create your own. Even if a statement doesn't seem to be true at the time you say it, keep saying it with feeling because it will attract to you what you desire. For example, an affirmation is "I am happy and my body is healthy in every way." The more you repeat statements of this kind, the more likely you are to experience it in your life. Make them positive, present tense, and in the first person. They should be simple and to the point. Then, repeat, repeat, repeat and believe, believe, believe. The best time to repeat affirmations is when the mind is receptive, such as when you are falling asleep, waking up, or around meditation.

BREATHING. We all breathe. There are so many different breathing techniques it's impossible to even begin to cover them here. Most people tend to breathe too shallow. When we do not get enough oxygen into our system, we feel more stressed and tired. The breath provides energy and relaxation to the muscles, even that pain in your neck or that hot flash needs some oxygen. Learning to breathe more deeply, especially if you are experiencing stress, will immediately bring oxygen to the muscles and allow you to relax. Here is a relaxation breath which works wonders on any kind of stress.

Relaxation Breath:

> Sit in a straight-backed chair with your feet flat on the floor. Be sure your back is straight and hands rested in your lap. Close your eyes as you inhale through your nose and count: one, two, three and four. Then pause or hold your breath as you count from one to seven. Then, exhale through your mouth as you count from one to eight. Use the count as a rhythm. Repeat four times. Notice how relaxed your muscles become and how quiet your mind becomes.

MEDITATION is stilling your body as well as your mind. Breathing and visualization are aspects of meditation, and there are many, many ways to meditate. For me, meditation is a special "time out," where I find a quiet spot to sit, rest quietly, and do nothing but clear my mind by focusing on a *mantra* (a word, sound, image or prayer). I recommend you learn meditation for enhanced results in all areas of health.

- Mantra Meditation – focus on *mantra* (a repetitive word, sound, image or prayer)
- Mindfulness Meditation – watching and/or counting your breaths
- Guided Meditation – you are guided through a relaxation imagery or visualization by a person or tape.

- Heart-Centered Meditation – focus at your heart level, and imagine sending love and healing to yourself, your family, and anyone else you choose.

There is no right or wrong way to meditate, however, meditation needs to be practiced regularly to achieve the best results. I begin each day with a meditation. You can too!

VISUALIZATION is a simple and powerful technique that you have used many times in your life whether you realize it or not. Visualization improves your imagination and creativity. Throughout this guide, visualizations, images, and pictures have been suggested for you to alleviate certain conditions. Since we think in pictures, it is important to have a clear picture of what you want, or what you want to achieve. Clear pictures, clear ideas, and clear feelings all help. For example, if you want to reduce a pain, take a few moments and breathe into the pain and feel it. It may seem more intense in that moment as you focus on it. Then, as you breathe, send conscious thoughts of healing light to your area of pain, imagine the light bringing comfort, soothing, and healing, and when breathing out, consciously "let go" of the pain. As you practice for several minutes, notice what happens.

You can do visualizations with your eyes closed and rested in a relaxed position either sitting or lying down. Visualization actually can be done anytime or anywhere. It is the intention and attention that you give it that makes it so powerful.

Any and all of these techniques can be used to relax. Once you start doing breathing, meditation, visualization, or affirmations regularly, you will look forward to them and begin to appreciate their magical effect. They all provide much more than just relaxation, they provide peace of mind and inner healing. A little time and effort now, will save you lots of time and trouble later. Remember, it's never too late to start.

Vitamins – Minerals – EFA'S

A good multiple vitamin and mineral supplement taken daily in addition to a healthy diet is important. Why? Because much of our food supply is grown in soils which are depleted of important minerals. U.S. Senate Document No. 264 (1936) contains information regarding the dietary deficiencies caused by food grown in soils depleted of certain minerals. In the absence of proper minerals, vitamins cannot adequately perform in the body either.

Because of inadequate soil, much fresh produce and whole grains lack the proper nutrients. *I heard that if you were to eat an apple off the tree in your grandparent's back yard fifty years ago, you would have to eat twenty-four apples today to get the same amount of nutritive value!* So, do yourself a favor, and take a vitamin and mineral supplement, and, yes, do eat an apple a day, unwaxed and organic if possible.

All vitamins and minerals are important, however, sometimes a little more of one specific vitamin or nutrient is needed. Many referrals to this are made throughout this guide. For now, I will cover the antioxidants and the essential fatty acids (EFA's) only.

Antioxidants are extremely important because they help scavenger and neutralize free radicals. Free radicals contribute to breakdowns in the body related to all illness, aging, and much more. Antioxidants are protective and keep the body strong. Antioxidants are often referred to as the ACES. Here they are:

Antioxidants

VITAMIN A/BETA–CAROTENE an antioxidant that helps maintain healthy skin, vision, hair, nails, teeth, and thought to be protective against cancer. Found in foods such as liver, eggs, carrots, sweet potatoes, cantaloupe, and papayas. Minimum amount needed is 8,000 mg/day, however other recommendations suggest 25,000 to 50,000 mg./day. Beta-carotene is considered safer than Vitamin A because it is converted into Vitamin A by the body when the organs are functioning properly.

VITAMIN C an antioxidant that humans cannot manufacture internally, so we must get it through the food we eat or take a supplement. Vitamin C promotes healthy cell membranes, gums, teeth, aids in production of collagen, and much, much more. It is found in citrus fruits, tomatoes, strawberries. Recommendations vary, however, usually 2,000 to 4,000 mg./day is a good start and more when you're ill. It's easy to know if you've taken too much Vitamin C because you will develop loose bowels. Should that happen, then just cut back on the amount you are taking. This should not occur at the levels mentioned here. It is best to take Vitamin C a couple times a day rather than all at once so the body can absorb it better. Whenever possible, choose one with Bioflavanoids.

VITAMIN E an antioxidant that protects tissues from oxidation and is significant in formation of red blood cells, helps with fibrocystic breasts, hot flashes, and heart disease. Found in vegetable oils, wheat germ, whole grains, nuts. 400 to 800 International Units are suggested, however, more may be required for certain conditions.

SELENIUM is also an antioxidant and a mineral that is shown to be helpful in preventing heart disease and cancer. Supplements are a better and more reliable source for selenium because selenium is found primarily in foods such as beef, pork, ham, and white bread, foods we need to eat in limited portions. However, fish is also a good source. Recommendation is to take between 50 to 200 micrograms per day. Vitamin E and selenium act synergistically and are good to take together.

Essential Fatty Acids & Omega 3 Oils

Essential Fatty Acids (EFA's) cannot be made by the body, and therefore, must be supplied through the diet. Although Americans eat a high-fat diet, it is the wrong kind of fat. The key is to lower "bad" fats that contribute to cholesterol and heart problems and eat "good" fats that are protective. These are the EFA's, and in particular Omega 3 oils.

The good fats and Omega 3's are mostly found in cold-water fish, like salmon and cod, but are also found in flax seed oil, evening primrose, and black currant oil. The EFA's have a beneficial effect on reducing blood pressure, aid in prevention of arthritis, reduce growth rate of breast cancer, lower cholesterol and triglyceride levels, and are helpful for eczema, psoriasis, arteriosclerosis, and more.

My recommendation is to use flax seed oil or flax seeds. Flax seed oil can be purchased in gel capsules or as a liquid oil. The oil can deteriorate so keep it in the refrigerator. Because it deteriorates very quickly in heat, do not cook with it. It can be used in dressings or drizzled over foods.

I like to use flax seeds. They are relatively inexpensive. The best way to use them is to grind them in a coffee grinder in order to break open the hard seedpod. Use it to sprinkle over cereal, salads, cottage cheese, etc. Again, keep the ground seeds in the refrigerator.

Sources for Omega 3's are:

- Flax seed oil
- Borage oil
- Black Currant oil
- Fish oils.

For additional information on other vitamins, minerals and nutrients refer to *Prescription for Nutritional Healing,* by James and Phyllis Balch.

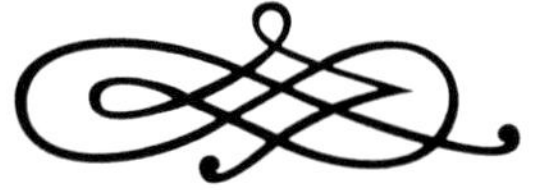

– Part IV –

Resources

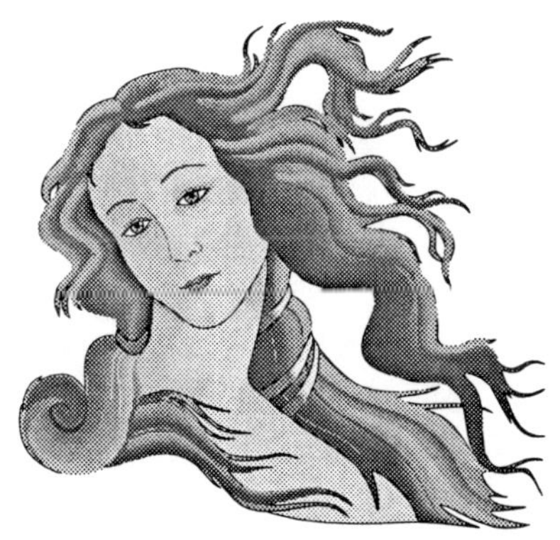

"I found this book to be very informative and useful on a variety of women's issues. Whenever I was looking for information on a specific topic, it was quite easy to find."

Kathy E., Age 52
Tai Chi Instructor and
Massage Therapist

Ten Tips To Empower Yourself

Here is my pep talk to you. Your actions are what will matter to you and your health in the end. Listen to the messages your body gives you daily, through every twinge, ache, pain, and more. Ask, question, research, and only decide when you feel clear and confident in the answer. You can do it!

1. **Change your PERCEPTION and MANAGE** your own health. Be more aware of your body, and especially the challenge of hormone balance throughout your life. As you change, the world changes with you. Allow any health experience to be a time of growth, wisdom, and self-empowerment.

2. **EXERCISE!** It's the best medicine. Do something every day whether it's walking, yoga, stretching, whatever you will do. Even five or ten minutes offer wonderful results. Notice how good you feel and how your body, mind, spirit, and emotions respond in positive ways.

3. Incorporate some type of **RELAXATION PROGRAM** on a regular basis and daily if possible. Breathing techniques, meditation, visualization, prayer, whatever you enjoy, and then choose the one you prefer. The easiest and surest way to stay cool, calm, collected, and healthy.

4. **DRINK PLENTY OF WATER DAILY.** If you have not done this before, NOW is the time. Drink at least eight 8 ounce glasses of water every day. This does not mean coffee, colas, teas, or juices. Plain, preferably filtered or purified, water is best. Drink upon rising and throughout the day between meals. Remember to drink only around one-half cup of liquid with meals, otherwise, too much liquid tends to dilute digestive juices.

5. **GIVE UP CAFFEINE,** especially coffee and soft drinks! Coffee and soft drinks stress the adrenal glands and rob the body of precious calcium. You need strong adrenals so they can do their job when the ovaries slow down. The

adrenals are an alternate source for producing hormones. Keep them happy. Try herbal teas or all natural coffee substitutes, such as Nature's Sunshine brand of instant Herbal Beverage, which is a very good coffee substitute.

6. **EAT A HEALTHY, OPTIMAL DIET.** (See guidelines in the "Nutrition" section.)

7. Have **GOOD ELIMINATION.** One good bowel movement a day is essential. Two or three are great! Toxins and excess estrogen are eliminated through waste. (See section on "Constipation").

8. **GET SUPPORT.** Share your feelings and talk to someone. Join a support group or start one of your own with friends. Expressing your feelings and concerns with others is very healing and empowering, plus you will learn from each other too.

9. **GET INFORMED.** Read books, articles, anything, and everything to teach yourself about your body, women's conditions, and alternative remedies. The "Suggested Reading List" at the end of this guide is a good place to start.

10. Chose an **OPEN-MINDED DOCTOR** and one who is sympathetic to your needs and desires. If you do not understand something, be sure to question him about it. Let him tell you about his remedies while you tell him about other more natural solutions, especially ones you've tried and that have worked for you. Someone has to do it!

Suggested Reading List

Reading is one of the best ways to educate yourself and gain more insight on any subject. Here's a few suggestions to get started.

What Your Doctor May Not Tell You About Menopause, John R. Lee, M.D. with Virginia Hopkins. Warner Books, Inc., New York, 1996. Basic information we can all use plus full explanation of progesterone and its roles.

What Your Doctor May Not Tell You About Premenopause, John R. Lee, M.D. with Jesse Heanley, M.D., Virginia Hopkins, Warner Books, Inc., New York, 1999.

Women's Bodies, Women's Wisdom, Christiane Northrup, M.D. Bantam Books, New York, 1994. Covers everything from diet, hormones, genetics, beliefs, and more.

The Wisdom of Menopause, Creating Physical and Emotional Health and Healing During the Change, Christiane Northrup, M.D., Bantam Books, New York, 2001.

Super Nutrition For Menopause, Ann Louise Gittleman, Pocket Books, New York, 1993. Nutritional approach to all conditions, plus good explanations of nutrients.

Hormone Book, Susan Love, Random House, New York, 1997. Offers the medical side as well as alternatives, herbs, homeopathics, and is good reading.

Menopausal Years: The Wise Woman Way, Susun Weed. Woodstock, NY, Ash Tree Publishing, 1992. Excellent reference for herbs, home remedies, and what to expect.

The Estrogen Decision, Susan M. Lark, M.D., Celestial Arts, Berkeley, California, 1995.

Hormone Replacement Therapy: Yes or No?, Betty Kamen, Ph.D., Nutrition Encounter, 1993

Menopause, Naturally, Preparing For the Second Half of Life, Sadja Greenwood, M.D. Volcano Press, Volcano, CA, 1984, 1989.

Menopause Without Medicine, Linda Ojeda, Ph.D., Hunter House, Alameda, California, 1995.

Smart Medicine for Menopause, Sandra Cabot, M.D., Avery Publishing Group, Garden City Park, New York, 1995.

The Natural Remedy Book For Women, Diane Stein, The Crossing Press, Freedom, California, 1992.

Resources

NATIONAL COMPOUNDING PHARMICIES

College Pharmacy
3505 Austin Bluffs Pkwy. Suite 101
Colorado Springs, CO 80918
1-800-888-9358
Website: www.collegepharmacy.com

Women's International Pharmacy
5708 Monona Drive
Madison, WI 53716
1-800-279-5708
Website: www.womensinternational.com

Women's International Pharmacy
12012 North 111th Ave.
Youngtown, AZ 85363
1-800-699-8143

Ask if there is a local
COMPOUNDING PHARMACY in your area.

SOURCES FOR SALIVA HORMONE TESTS

Aeron Lifecycles Lab	1933 David St., Suite 310 San Leandro, CA 94577 1-800-631-7900 Fax 510-729-0383
ZRT Laboratory	1815 NW 169th Place, Suite 5050 Beaverton, OR 97006 503-466-2445 Fax 503-466-1636 www.salivatest.com

All the hormones, including each of the estrogens, progesterone, testosterone, DHEA, adrenal hormones, and more can be tested by these labs. Contact them directly to get instructions, pricing, and a collection kit. Saliva tests are considered more accurate than blood tests for hormone levels.

SUGGESTED HERB & VITAMIN BRANDS

There are many more brands to choose from than are listed here. These are only a few. Many of these herbs can be found on the internet by doing a search for "herbs" or "vitamins."

Country Life
Crystal Star
Enzymatic Therapy
Ethical Nutrients
Nature's Life
Now
Rainbow Lights
Solaray
Twin Labs

TINCTURES

Gaia
Herb Pharm
Nature's Answer
Rainbow Lights

Most of these products are available at health food stores. Check in your local area.

SUGGESTED NAME BRAND PRODUCTS

Barleans – Flax Seed Oil
Found in most health food stores or visit website at www.barleans.com

Benefiber® – Sugar Free Soluble Fiber Supplement
Found in many drug stores

Floradex Liquid Herbal Iron
Found in most health food stores or call 800-446-2110

JuicePlus+® – Whole Food in Capsules
Not found in stores so contact local representative or visit website www.juiceplus.com

NSP (Nature's Sunshine Products)
Contact local NSP representative or locate NSP store in your area by calling 800-223-8225 or visit website at www.naturessunshine.com

PROGESTERONE CREAMS

Arbonne International – Multilevel Marketing Product
Contact local distributor in your area or visit website at www.arbonne.com

- Prolief – Progesterone cream
- PhytoProlief – Progesterone/Estrogen Herbs cream

Proprietary Blend Cream – Available only through Health Care Practitioners including the author (with consultation only)

- Progesterone cream
- Progesterone/Estriol cream
- Progesterone/Estriol/DHEA cream

Pro-Gest Products – Available Over The Counter

- Transitions for Health – Progesterone cream

OTHER RESOURCES

Curves For Women®, 30 Minute Fitness Centers
Phone 800-848-1096
Visit website at www.curvesforwomen.com

The Kegel Exerciser®, FDA Approved
Phone 866-953-4357
Visit website at www.apersonalsolution.com

Optimum Health Institute in San Diego, CA
Phone 800-993-4325
Visit website at www.optimumhealth.org

United Soybean Board for Recipes and Information
Phone 800-301-3153
Visit website at www.unitedsoybean.org

AROMATHERAPY

There are many different Essential Oil brands. A couple you may find easily include: AuraCacia, Nature's Alchemy, Tifferet, Tisserand, or Oshadhi. These may be found in many health food stores or spas, which may market other equally good brands. Also, you can do a search on the internet for "Aromatherapy."

References

Balch, James F. M.D. and Phyllis, C.N.C., *Prescription for Nutritional Healing,* Avery Publishing Group, Inc., Garden City Park, New York, 1990.

Cabot, Sandra, M.D., *Smart Medicine for Menopause,* Avery Publishing Group, Garden City Park, New York, 1995.

Coney, Sandra, *The Menopause Industry,* Hunter House, Alameda, CA, 1994.

Diamond, Harvey, *You Can Prevent Breast Cancer!,* ProMotion Publishing, San Diego, CA.

Epstein, Gerald, M.D., *Healing Visualizations, Creating Health Through Imagery,* Bantam Books, 1989.

Gittleman, Ann Louise, *Super Nutrition For Menopause,* Pocket Books, New York, 1993.

Gladstar, Rosemary, *Herbal Healing for Women,* Simon and Schuster, New York, 1993.

Greenwood, Sadja, M.D. , *Menopause, Naturally, Preparing For the Second Half of Life,* Volcano Press, Volcano, CA, 1984, 1989.

Hobbs, Christopher, *Vitex, The Women's Herb,* Botanica Press, Santa Cruz, CA, 1996.

Jacobowitz, Ruth S., *150 Most Asked Questions About Menopause,* Hearst Books, New York, 1993.

Kamen, Betty, Ph.D., *Hormone Replacement Therapy Yes or No?,* Nutrition Encounter, Novato, California, 1995.

Lark, Susan M. M.D., *The Estrogen Decision,* Celestial Arts, Berkeley, California, 1995.

Lavabre, Marcel, *Aromatherapy,* Healing Arts Press, Rochester, Vermont, 1990.

Lee, John R., M.D., with Hopkins, Virginia, *What Your Doctor May Not Tell You About Menopause,* Warner Books, Inc., New York, 1996.

Love, Susan, *Hormone Book,* Random House, Inc., New York, 1997.

Mindell, Earl, *Herb Bible,* Simon & Schuster/Fireside, New York, 1992.Northrup, Christiane, M.D., *Health Secrets For Women,* Phillips Publishing, Inc., 1995.

Northrup, Christiane, M.D., *Women's Bodies, Women's Wisdom,* Bantam Books, New York, 1994.

Page, Dr. Linda, *Healthy Healing Guide To Menopause & Osteoporosis,* Healthy Healing Publications, 1997.

Pedersen, Mark, *Nutritional Herbology,* Wendell W. Whitman Company, Warsaw, Indiana, 1994.

Pennington, Jean, A.T., *Food Values,* 15th edition, Harper Perennial, New York, 1989.

Rose, Jeanne, *The Aromatherapy Book,* North Atlantic Books, Berkeley, CA, 1992.

Royal, Penny C., *Herbally Yours, Sound Nutrition,* Hurricane, Utah, 1991.

Stein, Diane, *The Natural Remedy Book for Women,* The Crossing Press, 1992.

Tisserand, Maggie, *Aromatherapy for Women,* Healing Arts Press, Rochester, Vermont, 1988.

Weed, Susun, *Menopausal Years: The Wise Woman Way,* Woodstock, NY, Ash Tree Publishing, 1992.

Whitaker, Julian, M.D., *Dr. Whitaker's Guide to Natural Healing,* Prima Publishing, Rocklin, CA, 1996.

ARTICLES

Avila, Rafael "The Super Isoflavones," *Energy Times,* February 1997.

Brody, Jane E. "Selenium May Hold Several Benefits to Health," *San Diego Union Tribune,* February 26, 1997

Dranov, Paula, "Estrogen" *American Health,* December, 1996.

Fallon, Sally, M.A. and Enig, Mary, Ph.D. "Butter is Better," *Health Freedom News,* November/December 1995.

Fallon, Sally,M.A. and Enig, Mary, Ph.D. "Soy Products for Dairy Products?" *Health Freedom News,* September, 1995.

Kushi, et. al., "Physical Activity and Mortality in Postmenopausal Women," *The Journal of the American Medical Association,* April 23, 1997.

Lee, John, M.D. and Wright, Jonathan, M.D. "The Many Clinical Benefits of Natural Progesterone," *Life Enhancement,* February, 1997.

Liebman, Bonnie, Breast Cancer" *Nutrition Action Health Letter,* January/February, 1996.

Northrup, Christiane, M.D., "Oh, My Aching Breasts: What To Do About Mammary Soreness," *Health Wisdom for Women,* May, 1996.

Northrup, Cristiane, M.D., "Going With the Flow, What to do About Heavy Menstrual Periods," *Health Wisdom for Women,* June, 1996.

Rogers, Sherry A., M.D., "The Estrogen Answer" from the *Northeast Center For Environmental Medicine Health Letter,* Jan/Feb 1995.

Weil, Andrew, "Menopause Naturally," *Self Healing Newsletter,* April, 1997.

Weil, Andrew, "Reflexology Offers Whole-Body Benefits," *Self Healing Newsletter,* May, 1997.

VIDEOS

Veryl Rosenbaum, *Menopause Taking Charge,* Video II, Durango, CO 81302, 1-800-259-3172.

Dr. Alan Xenakis, *What Every Woman Should Know About Menopause,* Xenejenex Productions, 1993, 1-800-228-2495.

"If you want to see what
your thoughts were like yesterday,
look at your body today.
If you want to see what your
body will be like tomorrow,
look at your thoughts today."

Old Indian Proverb

Index

A

B

C